Manufacturing Bottleneck: Can We Afford the Future of Cell Therapy

Kinky

Table of Contents

Chapter 1: Introduction

1.1 Cell therapy manufacturing

Cell therapies are an emerging form of therapy, with the potential to cure a number of diseases. Due to their use of live cells, which can dynamically respond to cues, cell therapies have many advantages over other conventional non-cell-based therapies. As of February 2021, 28 cell therapies have received FDA approval, including mesenchymal stem cells to treat numerous diseases such as cardiovascular disease and graft-versus-host disease, as well as chimeric antigen receptor T cells to treat hematological malignancies [2]. In addition, over 1700 cell therapies are currently in clinical trials, 45% of which involve the use of T cells [2].

One major bottleneck that precludes the widespread clinical adoption of cell therapies, is the inability to reproducibly and economically manufacture them. Cell therapy manufacturing processes are complex and costly, making the scale-up of allogeneic cell products and the scale-out of autologous cell products, difficult. Manufacturing autologous cell therapies are especially complicated, because industrial manufacturing of these single-batch, patient-specific products cannot be modeled after established models for manufacturing and distributing conventional therapeutics, such as monoclonal antibodies [3].

The National Institute for Standard and Technology's (NIST's) National Cell Manufacturing Consortium (NCMC) developed a 10-year roadmap for cell therapy manufacturing entitled "Achieving Large-Scale, Cost-Effective, Reproducible Manufacturing of High-Quality Cells: A Technology Roadmap to 2025" that establishes key advances needed to increase the availability of cell-based technologies such as cell therapies [4]. As well as highlighting the need for reproducible cell therapy manufacturing processes, they also delineate many technological improvements required to improve various steps in the manufacturing process, including novel methods and devices to select the desired cells in an accurate and efficient manner during cell processing.

In this book we consider two emerging forms of cell therapy, organoid-based cell therapies, which require reproducible and scalable manufacturing, and adoptive cell therapies (ACT), which require simplified and cost-effective selection steps, in order to facilitate their clinical translation, and meet the potentially high demand in the future.

1.2 Organoids as a cell therapy

Three-dimensional cellular clusters, such as spheroids, in which cells simply aggregate together [5], or organoids, which self-organize and mimic the structure and function of native tissues [6], are commonly used for disease modeling and drug screening applications [7, 8], and are also an emerging form of cell therapy [9]. 3D cell culture has many advantages in comparison to traditional 2D cell culture, including providing a more physiological microenvironment for the cells to grow in, and allowing the formation of more native-like cell-cell, and cell-extracellular matrix (ECM) contacts [9]. As such, delivering cell therapies in the form of 3D cellular clusters, where the cells are within well-controlled microenvironments, can promote and maintain desired cellular functions within dynamic and complex environments in comparison to conventional cell therapies which consist of suspensions of single cells [10-15]. Organoid- and spheroid- based cell therapies have been assessed in pre-clinical studies for many therapeutic applications [9], including adipose-derived stem cell clusters to treat myocardial infarction [16], beta cell or islet cell organoids to treat Type 1 diabetes [17], and lung spheroids to treat pulmonary fibrosis [18]. More recently, 3D cell clusters have also been assessed in clinical trials worldwide, including for example Spherox, which are spheroids composed of autologous matrix-associated chondrocytes, to treat cartilage lesions [19]. As organoids are increasingly being explored for therapeutic purposes, there is increasing recognition of the unmet challenge in generating multicellular aggregates with high reproducibility and control. For example, as stated by Huch et al., [20] even though control over "organoid size, shape, cellular composition and 3D architecture [...] is essential in order to understand the mechanisms that underlie organoid development in normal and pathological situations, and to use them as targets for manipulation or drug testing", reproducibility has been cited as "the major bottleneck of current organoid systems".

A number of conventional methods to form 3D cell clusters exist, including spinner cultures [21], hanging drops [22, 23] and non-adhesive 96-well plates [24-27]. However, in addition to the lack of scalability, many of these methods also lack control and reproducibility, features which are especially important for use as a cell therapy. Alternatively, microtissues that are "cells in gels" [28-31] typically feature cells moving to pre-formed pores within a hydrogel scaffold, but the cells are limited in their ability to self-organize into desired structures [32], and the resultant gels exhibit variable structures and sizes dependent on the pores and may be undesired in the implanted site due to potential immunogenicity. More recently, methods to fabricate organoids based on micro-sized wells have faced challenges of either high adsorption (of steroid hormones, small molecules, and drugs [33, 34] for PDMS-based wells) or inefficient and harsh processes, usually involving vigorous pipetting or high-speed centrifugation, to separate and remove the cellular clusters from the microwells. Such procedures produce cellular clusters at a low yield and could damage cellular structures and function. Recognizing this limitation, other studies have proposed more complex methods to actively release cellular clusters from microwells [35-37]. As such, there still lacks reliable methods to generate organoids at high yield and with reproducibility and control over aggregate size and cellular organization, which is necessary to manufacture organoids for cell therapies.

1.3 Adoptive cell therapy to treat cancer

ACT is an emerging form of cancer immunotherapy which involves the delivery of autologous or allogeneic T cells, which are reactive against a target, such as tumor cells. Ultimately, the purpose of delivering T cells, is to enhance the cell-mediated adaptive immune response against the target.

1.3.1 Cell-mediated adaptive immune response

Typically, the cell-mediated adaptive immune response mobilizes host antigen-specific T cells to eliminate a target in the following manner [38]: 1. Programming of dendritic cells (DCs) : Immature DCs patrol the body, capturing and internalizing antigens that are processed into peptides and presented on major histocompatibility complex (MHC) class I or II molecules (referred to as pMHC). Activation of DCs by danger signals (such as pathogens or inflammatory stimuli) induces DC maturation into efficient antigen presenting cells through the increased transport and presentation of pMHC molecules, the up-regulation of co-stimulatory molecules, and DC migration to lymphoid organs [39]. 2. Activation of naive, antigen-specific T cells: In the T cell zone of lymphoid organs such as the spleen or lymph node, naive $CD4^+$ and $CD8^+$ T cells scan antigen-presenting DCs, to identify the DCs presenting pMHCs (MHCI for $CD8^+$ T cells, and MHCII for CD4$^+$ T cells) that are cognate to the T cell receptor (TCR) on the T cell. Binding between the cognate T cell and DC initiates T cell activation, which after 3-4 days results in the differentiation of naive T cells into effector or memory T cells [40]. Also, CD4$^+$ T cells can license DCs by signaling through CD40 on DCs and CD40L on CD4$^+$ T cells, which improves the ability of DCs to prime and activate CD8$^+$ T cells. 3. <u>T cells mediate effector responses against cells displaying target antigens:</u> Effector antigen-specific T cells then migrate to the relevant tissue and carry out their effector functions, whereby helper CD4$^+$ T cells (such as classical T-helper 1 or 2 cells) secrete a variety of cytokines which can help cytotoxic CD8$^+$ T cells eliminate target cells.

Despite the presence of the cell-mediated adaptive immune response (and other immune responses), tumors can still evade this response through a variety of immunosuppressive mechanisms [41, 42]. For instance, the tumor microenvironment consists of immunosuppressive regulatory T cells and myeloid-derived suppressor cells which can inhibit effector T cell function. Other mechanisms include abnormalities in antigen presentation and down-regulation of MHCI expression by tumor cells to evade T cells. Moreover, since some tumor antigens are also shared with healthy tissue, these antigens are considered to be self-antigens, and so the patient may not have T cells with a high reactivity to these shared antigens, due to the elimination of high affinity, self-antigen specific T cells during thymic selection [43].

In order to overcome these issues, ACT aims to infuse T cells, with targeted specificity to tumor antigens, into patients to promote anti-tumor activity.

1.3.2 Different forms of Adoptive T cell therapies

ACT involves delivering T cells (or other immune cells such as natural killer cells), to redirect the cell-mediated adaptive immune response against a particular target. Here, we briefly discuss the three main classes of adoptive T cell therapy: tumor-infiltrating lymphocytes (TILs), chimeric-antigen receptor (CAR) T cells, and TCR-engineered T cells.

TILs: Many tumors are enriched with tumor antigen-specific T cells that are unable to exert their functions due to chronic activation, and the presence of immunosuppressive molecules [44]. TILs are part of a highly personalized form of therapy which involves extracting tumor-reactive T cells from excised tumors, expanding them *ex vivo* and reinfusing them into the patient. Although not FDA-approved yet, TILs have demonstrated therapeutic efficacy in clinical trials against a number of cancers, including metastatic melanoma (complete tumor regression in 22% (20/93) of patients the majority of whom were still in complete remission for more than 3 years post-treatment [45]) and cervical cancer (objective tumor responses in 28% (5/18) of patients, two of which experienced complete remission, for at least 53 months post-treatment [46]).

CAR-T cells: CAR-T cells are T cells genetically modified with CARs, which are synthetic antigen receptors comprised of an extracellular monoclonal antibody to confer specificity of the T cell, transmembrane domain, costimulatory domain, and intracellular CD3 signaling domain [47]. Unlike conventional T cells, which are only reactive against antigenic peptides presented by an MHC molecule, CAR-T cells are reactive against protein antigens expressed on the cell surface in an MHC-independent manner. Since 2017, the FDA has approved four CD19-

targeting CAR-T cell products (tisagenlecleucel to treat acute lymphoblastic leukemia, axicabtagene ciloleucel to treat large B cell lymphoma, brexucabtagene autoleucel to treat mantle cell lymphoma, and lisocabtagene maraleucel to treat relapsed or refractory large B cell lymphoma [48]), and one B cell maturation antigen (BCMA)-targeting CAR-T cell therapy (idecabtagene vicleucel to treat multiple myeloma). Although CAR-T cells are very effective against certain B cell blood cancers, their efficacy in solid tumors remains limited [49]. This is likely because cell membrane-associated proteins that can be targeted by CARs comprise only 27% of the human proteome; thus, CAR-T cells would not be able to target the majority of cell surface markers [49]. Furthermore, there are few tumor-specific surface markers that can be targeted by CAR-T cells without causing on-target, off-tumor toxicities, since most surface proteins presented on tumor cells are also presented on healthy tissues [50]. In some cases, for example in CD19-targeting CAR T cell therapies that deplete both malignant and normal B cells, the elimination of healthy cells can be clinically managed, however, this is not always the case.

TCR-engineered T cells: TCR-engineered T cells are T cells that have been genetically modified with a TCR to redirect their reactivity to a new target (pMHC). Since TCRs can recognize peptides derived from the majority (73%) of the proteome, including cell surface, cytosolic, and intra-nuclear proteins, TCR-engineered T cells can target more antigens than CAR-T cells [49]. Although TCR-engineered T cells have not received FDA approval yet, they have been tested in numerous clinical trials [51], and their ability to target a greater breadth of antigens, including those that are tumor-specific, make them theoretically more effective against solid tumors in comparison to CAR-T cells [50].

1.3.3 Antigens that TCR-engineered T cells can be directed against

Tumors express a variety of different types of antigens which TCR-engineered T cells can be genetically modified to target. They are typically broadly classified as being tumor-associated antigens (TAA), which are presented by *both* tumor and healthy tissue, or tumor-specific antigens (TSA), which are *only* presented by the tumor [52]. Examples of TAAs include tissue differentiation antigens which are tissue-specific antigens that are expressed in both normal and tumor tissue, overexpressed tumor antigens which are expressed in normal tissue and overexpressed in tumors, and cancer/testis antigens. TAAs are more likely to be common across many patients, and so the same TCR could be engineered into multiple patients' T cells. However, a limitation of targeting TAAs is that as previously mentioned, since TAAs are considered self, the patients themselves may not have high affinity T cells specific to the TAAs due to tolerance mechanisms. Furthermore, although TCR-engineered T cells specific to TAAs have shown encouraging clinical results, they have also caused on-target/off-tumor toxicities by targeting healthy tissue presenting TAAs, and affinity-matured TCR-engineered T cells in particular have caused fatal off-target toxicities by cross-reacting with unrelated antigens [53]. In order to avoid on-target/off-tumor toxicities, T cells can be engineered with TCRs reactive against TSAs which include oncogenic viral antigens, derived from viruses that cause cancer, and neoantigens, arising from mutations in tumor cells and therefore only present on tumor cells. Neoantigens, in particular, are typically patient-specific, and since they are truly foreign to the body (not self-antigens), the host T cell repertoire should not be affected by central T cell tolerance, and so high-affinity T cells against neoantigens are more likely to be present within the patient [54].

1.3.4 Common methods used to select for antigen-specific T cells

A critical step in the development of T cell therapies such as TCR-engineered T cells with reactivity against the aforementioned types of antigens is the identification of (host or donor) antigen-specific T cells. T cell selection assays include conventional assays which identify activated T cells through ELISpot, intracellular cytokine staining or the upregulation of activation markers, as well as assays that assess TCR specificity, through the use of peptide-MHC multimers [55]. However, as stated by Yossef et al., "Effectively identifying and harnessing neoantigen-reactive T cells for patient treatment remains a challenge and it is unknown whether current methods to detect neoantigen-reactive T cells are missing potentially clinically relevant neoantigen reactivities" [56]. The same group further demonstrated that conventional screening technologies lack the efficiency to select all clinically relevant T cells. Others have similarly expressed doubt in the ability of existing technologies to select all antigen-specific T cells, for example, Danilova et al., [57] wrote "Based on these conventional assays, investigators have concluded that only a small number (generally <4) of potential [neoantigens] are recognized in a given cancer patient, even when there are hundreds identified by prediction algorithms in cancers with high mutational burden. A question remains as to whether the repertoire of functional [neoantigen]-specific T cells is in fact that limited or whether existing assays are not sensitive enough to identify larger repertoires. Thus, there is a need for new technologies to accurately select for rare, (neo)antigen-specific T cells, to potentially improve clinical outcomes. Furthermore, since neoantigens are typically patient-specific, the identification of neoantigen-specific T cells would have to occur at a personalized level (unlike TCRs reactive against TAAs, which are present in multiple patients and could potentially be obtained from a TCR library). As such, there is a need for simple technologies to accurately and efficiently enrich and select for rare, antigen-specific T cells, which could be easily scaled-out to facilitate large-scale manufacturing.

1.4 Overview of work

The goal of this work is to develop new technologies to ensure reproducibility and scalability in cell therapy manufacturing, and to streamline critical processes, to reduce costs and save time. Ultimately, we demonstrate the use of three different types of technologies: hydrogels (**Chapter 2**), deep learning (**Chapter 3**) and microfluidics (**Chapter 4**), to reduce the complexity of cell therapy manufacturing, and help facilitate their clinical translation.

The contents of this book are organized in the following manner:

Chapter 1: Introduction

Chapter 2: Sacrificial scaffolds to reproducibly fabricate pre-vascularized organoids to treat hindlimb ischemia

In Chapter 2, we demonstrate the use of an alginate microwell-based scaffold to fabricate pre-vascularized organoids comprised of endothelial cells and mesenchymal stem cells in a scalable and reproducible manner. We demonstrate the ability to control organoid size and structure depending on the cell types used, ratio of cells, or size of the microwells. We also assess the functional activity of the pre-vascularized organoids to restore blood perfusion in a mouse model of hindlimb ischemia. Finally, we develop methods to improve the scalability of alginate scaffold production by making the process more automatable. Ultimately, this chapter demonstrates the ability to use the alginate microwell platform technology to improve the manufacturing of vascularized organoids for cell therapies.

My role in this work was to verify the reproducibility of the hEC:mMSC organoids, fabricate the mEC:mMSC organoids and perform the *in vivo* study to assess their ability to restore functional recovery in a mouse model of hindlimb ischemia. I also modified the alginate scaffold production protocol to improve its automatability.

This work is ongoing, with part of it resulting in a co-first author publication: N.S. Rossen*, **P.N. Anandakumaran***, R. zur Nieden*, K. Lo, W. Luo, C. Park, C. Huyan, Q. Fu, Z. Song, R.P. Singh-Moon, J. Chung, J. Goldenberg, N. Sampat, T. Harimoto, D. Bajakian, B.M. Gillette, S.K. Sia, (2020) Injectable therapeutic organoids using sacrificial hydrogels. iScience. (*denotes equal contribution)

Chapter 3: Rapid video-based deep learning of cognate versus non-cognate T cell – DC interactions

In Chapter 3, we develop and demonstrate the use of a trained deep learning model to rapidly and accurately classify videos of antigen-specific T cells based on their distinct interaction dynamics with cognate DCs, in comparison to interactions between non-cognate T cells and DCs. We demonstrate both experimental (addition of anti-CD40 antibodies) and computational (channel thresholding) improvements in methodologies, which significantly improved the model's accuracy. The end product is a trained deep learning model that can accurately classify cognate versus non-cognate T cell – DC interactions within only 20-80 minutes of interactions, and that can generalize well to different types of high and low affinity CD8$^+$ T cells. This algorithm may be used to identify cognate T cell–DC interactions to gain a deeper understanding of adaptive immunity and progression of diseases such as cancer and autoimmune diseases, or it could be incorporated into a cell sorting device to select, or enrich for, rare antigen-specific T cells for TCR-engineered T cell therapies.

My role in this work was idea conception, data collection, processing and analysis, as well as developing, training, and testing the deep learning model.

This work is completed, and a first author publication has been submitted to Scientific Reports: **P.N. Anandakumaran**, A Ayers, P Muranski, R.J. Creusot, S.K. Sia, (2021) Video-based deep learning of spatiotemporal T cell – dendritic cell interactions to classify antigen-specific cells. (Submitted).

Chapter 4: Microfluidic artificial lymph node to select antigen-specific T cells.
In Chapter 4, we develop a flow-through, lymph node inspired microfluidic device to select antigen-specific T cells based on their interaction dynamics with DCs, for downstream use in adoptive cell therapies. By flowing T cells through 3D networks of antigen-presenting DCs and leveraging the ability of antigen-specific T cells to make long-lasting, stable interactions with cognate DCs, we can trap antigen-specific T cells within the device, similar to how the T cell zone of the lymph node mediates the high-throughput selection of antigen-specific T cells. Development of this device involved optimizing for a number of design challenges, including the 3D printing protocol for fabricating the microfluidic devices with the appropriate feature sizes

and the creation of the 3D DC scaffold, as well as optimizing the adhesion of DCs to the microcarrier beads (MCs), the viscosity of the media that the DC-coated MCs were suspended in, and the flow rate with which the MCs are injected. Using agent-based simulations and experiments, we demonstrate the ability to preferentially select antigen-specific T cells in comparison to non-specific T cells in a one-compartment device, which can be easily scaled up to multiple compartments, to test T cell reactivity against multiple antigens.

My role in this work was idea conception, development and testing of the computational models, design, fabrication and testing of the device, and data analysis.

This work is ongoing, with a planned publication upon completion.

Chapter 5: Conclusions

Appendix A: Soft medical microrobots: Design components and system integration

In Appendix A, we discuss four key design elements of soft medical microrobots: locomotion, feedback control, functionality, and biocompatibility, and the need to integrate these elements to develop functional microrobots with clinical utility.

This work resulted in a co-first author review paper: R.D. Field*, **P.N. Anandakumaran***, S.K. Sia, (2019) Soft medical microrobots: Design components and system integration. Applied Physics Reviews. (*denotes equal contribution)

Chapter 2: Sacrificial scaffolds to reproducibly fabricate pre-vascularized organoids to treat hindlimb ischemia

2.1 Background

Pre-vascularized 3-dimensional multicellular clusters [58-60], which behave as vascularization units, have numerous translational applications, including the vascularization of tissue-engineered organs [61], and the treatment of cardiovascular diseases where angiogenesis is required, such as peripheral artery diseases and myocardial infarction [9]. Pre-vascularized cell aggregates can exert their therapeutic effects through integration of the tubular structures formed by endothelial cells (ECs) within the clusters with surrounding blood vessels, or by providing paracrine support through the secretion of pro-angiogenic factors by cell types such as mesenchymal stem cells (MSCs). Theoretically, their pre-vascularized nature is therapeutically beneficial in comparison to single cells, which would have to organize *in vivo,* thereby requiring more time to re-establish vascularization. Furthermore, the single cells could die from prolonged deprivation of oxygen and nutrients before they form the desired blood vessels and anastomose with host vasculature [62-64]).

However, for clinical uses, the pre-vascularized multicellular clusters must be manufactured in a reproducible manner to achieve consistent results, and they must be fabricated at scale, to produce enough for a single patient (if autologous cells), or for multiple patients (if allogeneic cells). Although different approaches have been used to fabricate various types of cellular clusters, many methods are inherently low-throughput and thereby limited in their scalability, nor are they amenable to gentle harvesting (Table 2.1). Furthermore, in terms of pre-vascularized spheroids or organoids in particular, many conventional methods, as well as specialized assays, lack demonstrated reproducibility and control over size and shape (Table 2.2).

Table 2.1. Advantages for different cell aggregation production methods

Cell Aggregate Production Method	High throughput	Output (no. of cell aggregates)	Easy automation (liquid handling in all steps)	Continuous observation	Easy harvesting	Reference
Hanging drops	-	60 to 384 per culture plate	+	-	+	[22, 65, 66]
Spinner culture	+	1,000s per spinner flask	+	-	+	[21]
Microwells	+	1,000s per mold	-	+	-	[13, 58, 67-69]
Non-adhesive 96 well plate	-	96 per culture plate	-	+	-	[24, 26, 27]
Sacrificial hydrogel microwells	++	10,000s per mold	+	+	+	Current study

Table 2.2: Reproducibility and control of vascularized organoids

Method for producing vascularized organoids	Control over size in cited study	Control over shape in cited study (circularity)	Reference
Hanging drop	Yes	High	[66]
Microwells	No	High	[58]
Non-adhesive 96 well plate	No	Medium	[27]
Thermoresponsive hydrogel sheets	Yes	Medium	[70]
Cells embedded within gels	No	Low	[71]
Sacrificial hydrogel microwells	Yes	High	Current study

Here, we take advantage of the dynamic responsiveness of hydrogels, to fabricate sacrificial alginate microwell scaffolds in which we can grow organoids, and then harvest them in a gentle manner simply by uncrosslinking the hydrogel. We specifically use the alginate microwell scaffolds to reproducibly, and controllably generate pre-vascularized organoids composed of ECs and MSCs. We then gently harvest the organoids and demonstrate their use as a cell therapy to treat a mouse model of peripheral artery disease (PAD) [72-76], the most severe form of which is critical limb ischemia (CLI), which often leads to amputations, due to the inability of surgical treatments such as stent placement or vascular bypass to re-establish microvasculature. Finally, we also modify the protocol to fabricate the alginate scaffold to make it more automatable, so that it could potentially be fabricated by an automated pipetting robot, and produced at scale. These sacrificial alginate scaffolds can be used to improve the manufacturing of various types of organoids for cell therapies, by generating them in therapeutic quantities, without disrupting their architectures, and reproducibly, in terms of size and organization.

2.2 Methods

2.2.1 Fabrication of sterile alginate microwells

A PDMS negative mold was previously fabricated by casting PDMS into an SU-8 (SU-8 3050, Microchem) master mold. The PDMS molds were made hydrophilic by plasma cleaning, and then autoclaved, moved to the biosafety cabinet, rinsed in PBS and filled with ~30 μL of autoclaved 7.5% (w/v) alginate (Sigma Aldrich) using positive displacement pipettes. A 6000 Da MWCO dialysis membrane was then placed over the alginate, and a glass slide was used to flatten the membrane and remove any excess alginate. 2 mL of 60 mM calcium chloride was pipetted on top of the membrane to enable the slow diffusion of calcium ions into the alginate in order to enable crosslinking. After around 1.5 hours of crosslinking, the calcium chloride solution was removed, the dialysis membrane was carefully peeled off of the PDMS/alginate wells, and each crosslinked alginate scaffold was carefully peeled out. Each scaffold was placed in one well of a 24-well plate (with the open microwells facing up) with 1.8 mM $CaCl_2$, and stored at 4°C overnight.

2.2.2 Uncrosslinking of sacrificial alginate

To determine the length of time required to uncrosslink the microwells, 7.5% w/v alginate microwell scaffolds were fabricated as described in the previous section, and stored in 1.8 mM $CaCl_2$ overnight. The following day, the scaffolds were transferred to pre-weighed, individually cut wells (from a 24-well plate), excess $CaCl_2$ was removed, and the initial mass of the scaffolds was measured. We then added 1 mL of PBS, 0.5% w/v sodium citrate, or 5% w/v sodium citrate to the well, and after 1 minute the excess supernatant was removed, the remaining alginate scaffold was weighed, and a fresh solution of PBS, 0.5% sodium citrate or 5% sodium citrate was added. This was repeated until the alginate microwell scaffold was fully uncrosslinked.

2.2.3 Cell sources

GFP-expressing human umbilical vein endothelial cells (hECs, Angio-Proteomie) were cultured in Endothelial Growth Medium 2 (Promocell). Mouse endothelial cells (mECs, Cell Biologics) were cultured in Complete Mouse Endothelial Cell Media (Cell Biologics). RFP-expressing mouse mesenchymal stem cells (mMSCs) (Cyagen) were cultured in DMEM with 10% fetal bovine serum (FBS) and 1% Penicillin-Streptomycin (P/S) (all from LifeTechnologies). All cells were gently passaged at 70-80% confluency, using TrypLE (LifeTechnologies) for the MSCs, and using 0.25% trypsin-EDTA solution for the ECs. The ECs were cultured until passage 6 and mMSC until passage 8. The cells were cultured in an incubator at 37°C and with 5% CO_2.

2.2.4 Fabrication of organoids

ECs and MSCs were harvested from flasks, counted and prepared at the desired ratio of ECs to MSCs, at a final concentration of 25×10^6 total cells/mL. Simultaneously, the 1.8 mM $CaCl_2$ solution that the alginate microwells were stored in was removed, and replaced with 1mL of maintenance media (full EC media without VEGF and EGF), and the microwells were incubated at 37°C and 5% CO_2 to equilibrate for at least 20 minutes.

20 μL of the cell suspensions was then pipetted onto alginate molds of 100, 200 and 400 μm microwell size using a positive displacement pipette. The wells were then moved to the incubator to allow the cells to settle at the bottom of the microwells for 20 minutes, after which another 1mL of maintenance media was added to each well. The organoids were cultured in maintenance media or the first 4 days of culture, and in a vascularizing media (full EC media with VEGF and EGF) for the remaining 4 days of culture, with media changes every other day. This total cell number (0.5×10^6) was selected because it is appropriate for all three microwell sizes, in terms of even cell distribution, and for forming a single organoid.

2.2.5 Harvesting of organoids

To collect the organoids, the alginate hydrogel was uncrosslinked [77]. For this, the culture medium of the organoids was replaced with 5% w/v sodium citrate solution for approximately 20 minutes. This chelator uncrosslinked the alginate, and allowed for resuspension of the organoids in a desired medium. Organoids were then centrifuged at 300 rpm for 5 minutes and the organoid pellet was carefully collected for further use.

2.2.6 Mice

All animal procedures were approved by the Columbia University Institutional Animal Care and Use Committee (IACUC) and all experiments were performed in accordance with relevant guidelines/regulations. C57BL/6J (B6) mice were purchased from The Jackson Laboratory (Bar Harbor, Maine).

2.2.7 Hindlimb ischemia surgery

Surgical procedures to induce hindlimb ischemia in B6 mice were conducted as described previously [78]. Briefly, ischemia was induced in the right hindlimb of the mouse by ligation and excision of the femoral artery between the distal side of the deep femoral artery bifurcation and the proximal side of the saphenous/popliteal bifurcation. The mice were anesthetized with isoflurane and maintained on a warmed surface. Intravenous injection of Buprenorphine and Carprofren, for analgesia, and saline, for increased hydration, were administered pre-operatively. Mice were positioned in dorsal recumbency with their hindlimbs externally rotated. Lidocaine, for local anesthesia, was administered subcutaneously at the shaven surgical site, which was subsequently sterilized with 70% ethanol and iodine. A skin incision was made over the femoral artery beginning at the inguinal ligament and continued caudally to the popliteal bifurcation. The femoral artery was isolated from the femoral vein and nerve bundle, and the femoral artery was doubly ligated and excised from the distal site of the deep femoral artery bifurcation to the saphenous and popliteal bifurcation. Immediately following femoral artery ligation, 0.1mL volume of organoids (corresponding to a total of 2×10^6 cells in saline), a single cell suspension of ECs and MSCs (at a 1:1 ratio corresponding to a total of 2×10^6 cells in saline), or saline alone were injected into the semimembranosus muscle at four sites around the injured site. The incision was closed with 4-0 nylon suture. Note that the 1:1 mEC:mMSC organoids were grown in the 200 μm alginate scaffolds, and were collected on day 4. Body temperature was maintained with heating pads until the animals recovered from surgery and were ambulatory. Animals were housed separately and closely monitored. The animal procedures were approved and carried out in accordance to local regulations and authorities. The surgeries were conducted in aseptic technique.

2.2.8 Laser speckle contrast imaging (LSCI) to measure perfusion

LSCI was used to measure perfusion of the injured and naive limbs on Day 0, 1, 2, 3, 5, 7, 9, 11 and 14 post-surgery. A LSCI system was built [79], consisting of a 810 nm infrared laser diode, a beam expander and a CCD camera with a band-pass filter. The mice were anesthetized with isoflurane and placed in sternal recumbency with the hindlimb stretched out behind them exposing the plantar surface of the hind paws. For each measurement, 40 consecutive images were obtained and the spatial speckle contrast was estimated from a 7x7 window of pixels [80]. Average hindlimb perfusion was determined for an anatomical defined region of the foot – the plantar surface of the hind paw spanning the digital, metacarpal and carpal pads. The calculated perfusion was expressed as a ratio of the mean perfusion of the planter surface of the right (ischemic) to the left (control) hindlimb.

2.3 Results

2.3.1 Fabrication of alginate microwell scaffolds

The use of alginate as a sacrificial scaffold to generate organoids was inspired by the use of

sacrificial materials in the micromachining of microelectromechanical systems (MEMS) to

release patterned metals or semiconductors from a substrate (Fig 2.1a). Hydrogels have also been

previously used to generate organoids due to the non-adhesiveness of specific hydrogels, which

facilitates cellular interactions, and contraction into spheroids and organoids [58, 68]. Alginate in

particular can alter the crosslinking state through the addition of calcium or a chelator [81-84],

which we sought to take advantage of, to release the organoids from the scaffold without

significantly disrupting its structures or underlying cell function [77]. Briefly, we deposit the

sacrificial material (alginate), create the sacrificial structure (alginate microwell scaffold) by

crosslinking the alginate in its patterned state, deposit cells on top to allow cellular self-

organization to take place, and remove the sacrificial layer by adding a chelator (5% w/v sodium

citrate) (Fig 2.1a). We demonstrate that the alginate microwell scaffold can be completely

uncrosslinked within ~12 minutes of incubation with a 5% sodium citrate chelator, thereby

releasing the organoids into solution, which can be collected for downstream manipulation (Fig

2.1b).

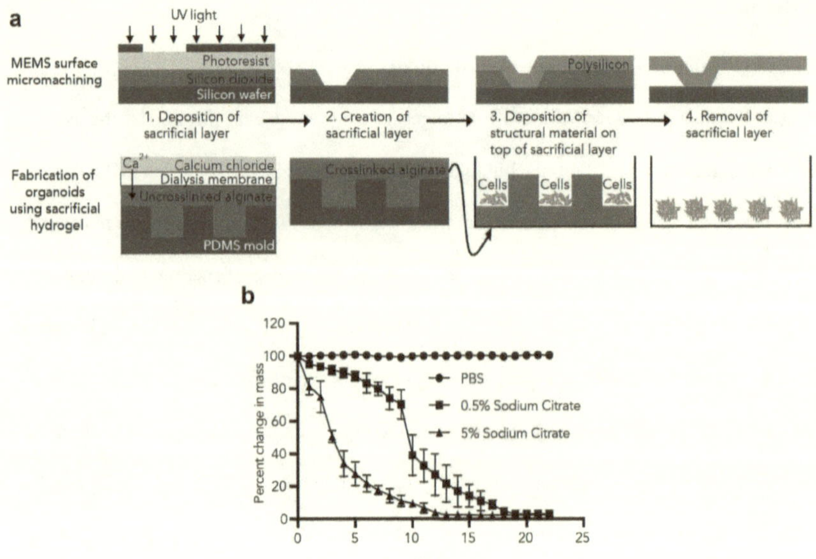

Figure 2.1: Schematic diagram of method of using sacrificial hydrogels to produce therapeutic organoids. (a) Schematic demonstrating the parallels between the surface micromachining method to fabricate MEMS devices such as a microcantilever (top) and the use of sacrificial alginate microwells to fabricate organoids (bottom), both of which use a sacrificial layer (blue) to fabricate the final structure (red). (b) Time required to completely uncrosslink alginate microwells following incubation with different concentrations of a chelator (sodium citrate) by measuring the percent change in mass over time (n=3, mean ± standard deviation).

The schematic diagram in Fig 2.2 zooms into the microwells within the scaffold, in which single cell suspensions of ECs and MSCs are seeded to induce cellular organization into pre-vascularized organoids, which can be harvested by uncrosslinking the alginate scaffold, and then injected *in vivo*. Each step is simple, can be conducted with sterile liquid handling, and can be automated.

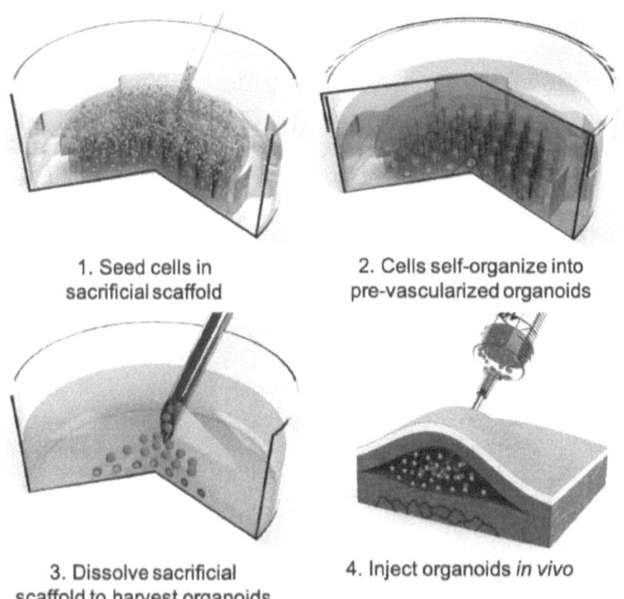

Figure 2.2: Schematic diagram of the microwell structures within the alginate scaffolds, where single ECs (green) and MSCs (red) self-organize into pre-vascularized organoids, which can then be easily harvested and injected *in vivo*.

2.3.2 Controllable, reproducible and scalable formation of pre-vascularized organoids grown in the alginate microwell scaffolds

We can also use the scaffolds to control the organoids in terms of size and structure. Using

scaffolds with 100, 200, or 400 μm diameter microwells, we can control the number of cells that

could aggregate into a single organoid, and hence, the organoid size (Fig 2.3a). In all cases,

although the human ECs (hECs) and mouse MSCs (mMSCs) were randomly distributed in the

wells on day 0, they aggregated into compact organoids by day 4 (The interactions between the

two cell types, despite originating from different species, is likely due to intercellular E-cadherin

interactions, which can cross-react between species [85, 86]). Varying the size of the microwells

(100, 200, and 400 μm diameter) yielded hEC and mMSC organoids of three different sizes

(39±3 µm, 71±5 µm, and 82±7 µm diameter, respectively). Also, we quantitatively analyzed the formation of organoids for cultures containing co-cultures with hEC:mMSC ratios of 1:3, 1:1, and 3:1. For the majority of the conditions, the ECs migrated towards the center of the organoid. However, we could further control organoid structure using the microwell size or ratio; for example, the co-cultures in 100-µm microwells did not form a distinct center, likely due to insufficient numbers of cells. Fig 2.3b quantifies the radius of the smallest circle that encompasses the MSCs or ECs in organoids formed in the 200 µm scaffolds. The decrease in radius is associated with the formation of compact organoids, and the small error bars further demonstrate the reproducibility in terms of size.

Also, in order to facilitate the clinical translation of these organoids by easily scaling up organoid production, alginate scaffolds of various sizes were fabricated: 15.6 mm-diameter inserts containing >1000 microwells (fits in a well of a 24-well plate), 22.1-mm inserts containing >3000 microwells (fits in a 12-well plate), and a 60-mm diameter insert containing >30,000 microwells (fits in a 60-mm culture dish) (Fig 2.3c). This demonstrates the scalability of this method.

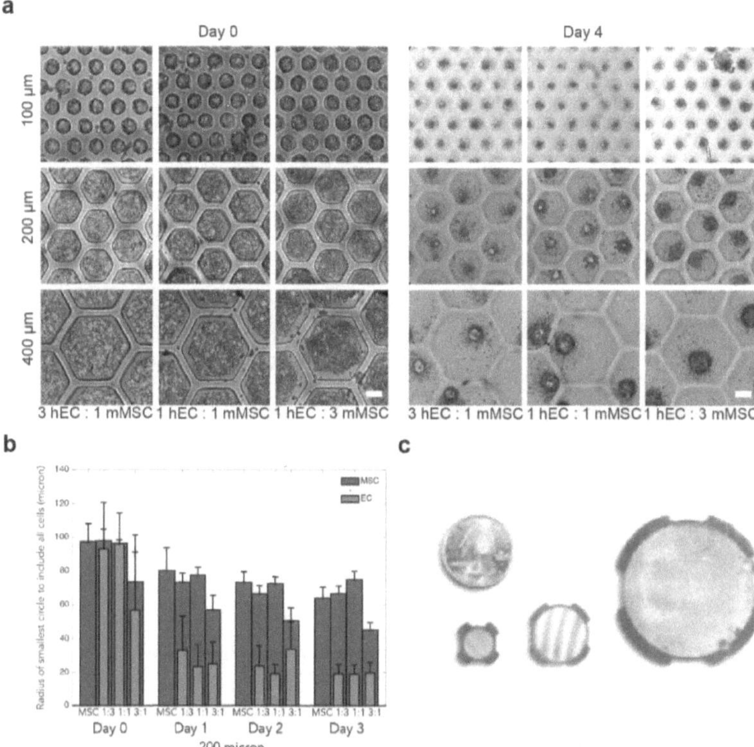

Figure 2.3: Production of reproducible organoids comprised of hECs (green) and mMSCs (red) (a) Images of hEC and mMSC organoids cultured in maintenance media at varying ratios of hECs to mMSCs, and in microwells with varying diameters, at day 0 and day 4. (b) Quantitative analysis of cell aggregation into organoids over time in 200 μm microwells, as measured by the radius of the smallest circle that can contain all MSCs (red) or all ECs (green) (n > 20). (c) Pictures of three alginate microwells constructs for inserts into 24-well plates, 12-well plates or 60-mm dishes with the capacity to produce 24 x 1000, 12 x 3000 or 30,000 organoids respectively.

2.3.3 Pre-vascularized organoids as a cell therapy to treat a mouse model of hindlimb ischemia

Since we were interested in assessing these pre-vascularized organoids in a mouse model of hindlimb ischemia, we fabricated organoids composed of mouse ECs (mEC) and mMSCs at ratios of 1:1 and 1:10 in the 200 μm diameter microwells (Fig 2.4a). The resulting organoids were reproducible within each of the conditions, however, we found that the 1:1 ratio resulted in organoids consisting of two distinct but fused structures, while the 1:10 ratio resulted in organoids where the ECs migrated to the center, similar to the structure observed in the hEC:mMSC organoids. This was especially interesting given the 1:1 hEC:mMSC organoids more robustly formed the core-shell structure than the 1:10 hEC:mMSC organoids.

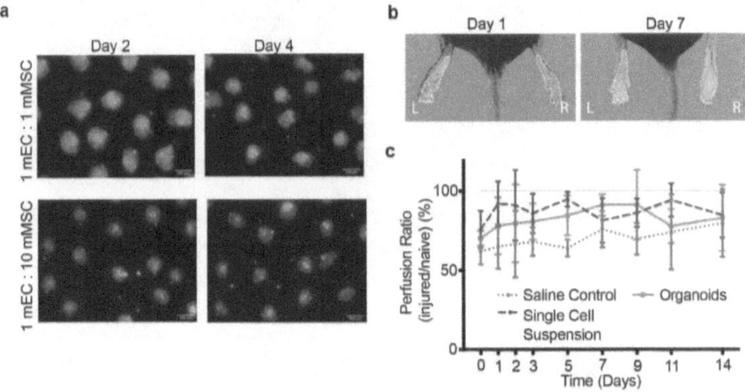

Figure 2.4: Functional recovery of murine ischemic hindlimb injury following delivery of pre-vascularized organoids comprised of mECs (green) and mMSCs (red). (a) Images of mEC and mMSC organoids cultured in maintenance media at varying ratios, in 200 μm microwells at day 2 and day 4. (b) Representative images of blood perfusion in the hindlimbs measured with LSCI for the organoid group. (c) Quantification of blood perfusion through hindlimbs expressed as a ratio of the mean perfusion of the right (ischemic) foot to the left (control) foot following delivery of 1:1 mEC:mMSC organoids (cultured for 4 days) (n=5), single cell suspension of mEC and mMSCs (n=3), or saline (n=5). (mean ± standard deviation).

We then conducted an *in vivo* study to assess the functional capacity of the mEC and mMSC organoids to restore blood perfusion, and improve the therapeutic outcomes in a murine model of hindlimb ischemia, in comparison to a single cell suspension of ECs/MSCs, and saline. Hindlimb ischemia was induced in the right limb via ligation and excision of the femoral artery between the distal site of the deep femoral bifurcation and the popliteal/saphenous bifurcation. We originally chose this surgical model as it consistently achieved reduced perfusion in the distal hindlimb, and was more reproducible and better represented chronic manifestations of atherosclerotic disease than more severe hindlimb ischemia models [87]. Immediately post-surgery, the various treatments were intramuscularly injected into the hindlimb at 4 sites, taking advantage of the robustness of the organoids to shear stress, and thereby obviating invasive surgery [88]. Note that the organoids treatment were composed of the 1:1 mEC:mMSC organoids despite the absence of the core-shell structure because it was unknown whether the core-shell structure was required for functionality, and also because we did not want to inject overwhelmingly more MSCs than ECs into the mice.

Blood perfusion was visualized and measured close to the planar surface of the paw using laser speckle contrast imaging (LSCI) (Fig 2.4b), which can image perfusion in microvasculature within 300 μm of the skin surface, and provide accurate relative measurements of velocity of blood flow [89]. We also used LSCI to ensure all of the mice were injured to the same degree, and to ensure fair comparisons between the different mice and different groups. In fact, one mouse from the organoid treatment group, and one from the saline control group were excluded from analysis because they were not injured to the same degree as the remaining mice. In the remaining mice, the aforementioned femoral artery ligation and excision in the right hindlimb induced ischemia and limited perfusion, as confirmed by the reduced perfusion ratio on day 0 immediately post-surgery, as measured by LSCI (Fig 2.4c).

In general, both the single cell and organoid treatments resulted in rapid recovery of blood perfusion in comparison to the saline control, which took more time (Fig 2.4c). However, there were little differences between the single cell and organoid treatments. This lack of difference could be attributed to a number of reasons, such as the mild nature of the ischemic injury. In this mild injury model, since mice that only received saline eventually fully recovered to the same degree as both treatment groups, the presence of the exogenous cells could accelerate recovery, simply by providing paracrine support to endogenous cells. By inducing a more severe ischemic injury, it is possible that cell replacement would be the dominant form of recovery, in which case the pre-vascularized nature of the organoids would be more beneficial in inducing recovery than single cells, which would first need to organize themselves *in vivo*, thereby lagging behind the organoids. Alternatively, culturing the organoids for more time *in vitro*, to allow the organoids to further organize and mature prior to *in vivo* delivery, could also improve recovery in comparison to single cells.

2.3.4 Modifying alginate scaffold fabrication to be more automatable

Finally, given the ability of this sacrificial scaffold system to improve the manufacturing of organoid-based cell therapy in terms reproducibility and scalability, we sought to also improve the fabrication of the scaffolds themselves, to make it more automatable. In particular, we modified the protocol such that it could potentially be automated by a pipetting robot, such as the one offered by Opentrons, which is a low-cost, open-source automated pipetting robot which moves a pipette in the x, y, z directions, and then applies a force on the pipette in the +z and -z direction to eject and draw liquids, respectively. Although the protocol for fabricating the alginate scaffolds was simple, there were two more challenging steps, which required user input and would be difficult to automate in the current state: placement of the dialysis membrane, and removal of the scaffolds from the PDMS mold after crosslinking. Placement of the membrane requires carefully grasping it with forceps, and slowly placing it on top of the alginate, without creating any bubbles in the alginate, and then scraping a glass slide across the membrane to remove any excess alginate, without moving the membrane itself.

In order to overcome the difficulties associated with placement of the dialysis membranes, we first attempted to switched from external gelation, which occurs when the calcium ions diffuse from the outside to the inside of the alginate, to internal gelation which involves the release of the calcium ions from within the alginate [90]. As such, we thought internal gelation could be a good alternative, because it does not require an externally placed dialysis membrane and calcium chloride, and rather involves mixing alginate with calcium carbonate and glucono delta-lactone to internally crosslink the alginate. However, the internally crosslinked alginate microwells were not homogeneously crosslinked, nor did they have the appropriate mechanical properties required to remove the microwells from the PDMS molds. Thus, internal gelation was not an appropriate solution here.

In order to facilitate membrane placement and removal of excess alginate, and to make this step automatable by a pipetting robot, we instead used dialysis inserts. The dialysis inserts are easier to handle than membranes alone, calcium chloride can be directly placed into the insert without spilling over, and excess alginate can be easily removed by simply pressing down on the plastic part of the insert. Furthermore, due to the close contact between the insert and the alginate, once the alginate is crosslinked, it often peels out of the PDMS mold when the insert is removed. We also 3D printed a "pipette" which could open and close its arms around an insert when a force is applied to it in the +z or -z direction, respectively. Future work involves miniaturizing this pipette to be able to fit inside the holders of an Opentrons robot.

2.4 Discussion

For purposes of cell therapy, it is critical for clinical efficacy, process control, and regulatory approval, that cells introduced into the body are generated via tightly controlled processes and exhibit reproducible origin, size, and structure. Previous studies have observed that a "lack of control over the process is likely to underpin the variability in systems and experiments that, with few exceptions, does not allow [organoids] to yield their full potential", and the importance of achieving reproducible "organoid size, shape, cellular composition and 3D architecture" in future research on organoids as well as use for therapeutic purposes [20]. Compared to current organoid systems, our method can generate self-organized multicellular aggregates with high yield (Table 2.1), as well as high control and reproducibility (Table 2.2). In this study, sizes and internal architectures of the organoids were reproducible for different types of cells (MSCs and ECs of mouse and human origin), cell ratios, and microwell diameter sizes.

Also, an ideal method for generating organoids should be scalable and gentle. In the common hanging-drop method, 384 organoids could be produced in the area of an overall standard well plate (with the overall scalability limited by the number of wells [22]), whereas the smallest construct shown in Fig 2.3c produces 24,000 organoids in the same area with fewer steps needed (e.g. media-changing steps, one alginate dissolving step), all of which could be automated by liquid handling. The release of organoids is gentle even at a large scale, in contrast to vigorous pipetting or high-speed centrifugation for current microwell procedures. For cell therapy, it is important that the integrity of the cells be preserved (for example, a FDA guidance document points to the need "to preserve integrity and function so that the products will work as they are intended" [91]). Beyond cell therapy, large-scale and effective production of organoids could also support studies in developmental biology, cancer cell intravasation [24], and organ printing.

To conclude, here, we demonstrate the use of a sacrificial alginate microwell scaffold to reproducibly generate and harvest pre-vascularized EC-MSC organoids at scale. We also conducted an *in vivo* study in order to assess the ability of these organoids to restore blood perfusion in a mild mouse model of hindlimb ischemia. Although not significant, the organoids are trending towards restoring perfusion more rapidly than saline controls. However, suspensions of single cells resulted in similar levels of recovery as organoids. Future work will involve assessing the organoid functionality in a more severe model of hindlimb ischemia, with optimized dosage and *in vitro* culture conditions (further discussed below). However, regardless of the functional outcomes, we demonstrate that the sacrificial hydrogel scaffold is a platform technology that improves the manufacturability of organoid-based cell therapies, and which can be applied to many different types of organoid-based systems.

Chapter 3: Rapid video-based deep learning of cognate versus non-cognate T cell – dendritic cell interactions

3.1 Introduction

Interactions between cognate T cells and antigen-presenting DCs are a critical component of the cell-mediated adaptive immune response, and peripheral tolerance. Cognate interactions between the TCR on T cells and antigenic pMHC complexes on mature DCs results in T cell priming, which directs T cells to respond to a target in an antigen-specific manner, whereas cognate interactions between T cells and immature or tolerogenic DCs results in peripheral tolerance, to maintain homeostasis [92, 93]. For understanding disease progression, the absence of T cell priming by cognate DCs or other antigen-presenting cells (APCs) prevents immune-mediated control of tumors [94], while the inappropriate priming of self-reactive T cells by cognate DCs is involved in the initiation and/or progression of autoimmune diseases such as Type 1 diabetes [93]. As such, there is a need to classify cognate T cell – DC interactions to understand their role in T cell priming, adaptive immunity, tolerance, and disease pathogenesis.

The identification of antigen-specific T cells is also necessary for the development of adoptive cell therapies such as TCR-engineered T cell therapies, which involve the delivery of T cells reactive against particular antigens, such as tumor antigens in the context of cancer [95], viral antigens in the context of virus-related cancers such as Epstein-Barr virus-related lymphomas [96], and of recent interest, membrane, spike and nucleocapsid antigens in the context of SARS-CoV-2 [97]. ACT can also be adapted to autoimmune diseases such as Type 1 diabetes, by delivering antigen-specific regulatory T cells to suppress T cells reactive against beta cell-derived autoantigens [98]. Identification and characterization of antigen-specific T cells which express TCRs that are reactive against particular viral or tumor epitopes bound to MHC (pMHC) complexes remains a challenging task due to the vast TCR repertoire, of which only a few (~1 in 10^6 peripheral blood T cells) are specific for a given antigen [99, 100].

Table 3.1: Other methods used to classify antigen-specific T cells

Reference	Experimental setup	Classification method	Classification of	Time required to culture T cells	Enrichment via expansion	Limited to pre-defined peptide sequences
[101]	Bulk culture	Intracellular cytokine staining	T cell activation	6-24 hours	Yes	No
[102]	Bulk culture	Tetramers	TCR specificity	1 hour	Yes	Yes
[103]	Trapping of genetically modified cells in microdroplets	Increased fluorescence	T cell activation	9 hours	No	No
[104]	Flowing cells through microfluidic channel	Velocity differences	TCR-pMHC affinity	Seconds	Unlikely (N/A for the cell types currently used)	Yes
[105]	Biopsy samples	Deep learning of morphological variables from static images	Cognate T cell – DC interactions	12 hours of *in vivo* interactions	No	No
[106]	Bulk culture	Machine learning of autofluorescence lifetime	T cell activation	72 hours	No	No
Current study	Bulk culture	Deep learning of videos	Cognate T cell – DC interactions	20-80 minutes	No	No

A number of bulk [107, 108] and single cell [103, 109, 110] assays have been developed in order to identify antigen-specific T cells from the vast T cell repertoire *in vitro*. However, many of these require hours of co-culture between T cells and DCs (or other APCs) prior to classification or are limited to pre-defined peptide sequences (Table 3.1). Moreover, due to the rarity of antigen-specific T cells in the peripheral blood, many of these methods are not sensitive enough to use alone, and therefore require an enrichment step prior to selection. This enrichment step typically involves expanding T cells in bulk, in the presence of the antigens of interest for multiple weeks to specifically amplify the antigen-reactive T cells. For example, Stronen et al. [107] co-cultured peripheral blood mononuclear cells (PBMCs) with autologous monocyte-derived DCs presenting specific antigens for 26 days to expand out antigen-specific T cells, after which antigen-specific T cells were selected and sorted using pMHC multimers. However, this expansion step is time-consuming and can distort the T cell population, as not all T cells are equally capable of clonal expansion, and could result in the overgrowth of certain T cell clones over others. For example, Yossef et al. [56] clonally seeded 1.5×10^3 T cells at ~3 cells/well and cultured them under rapid expansion protocols for three weeks, and found that only 64 wells grew, which corresponded to a growth efficiency of only ~13%. Recently, antigen-specific T cells have also been enriched by selecting for T cells expressing specific surface markers, such as PD-1 [111], 4-1BB [112], or CD39 [113]. However, the sensitivity of these methods to enrich antigen-specific T cells is unknown [114]. Thus, there is a need for enrichment-free methods of T cell selection, or, if enrichment is necessary, there is a need for sensitive, expansion-free enrichment methods.

Deep learning is a subset of machine learning, which uses neural networks to learn abstract representations of data, and has been used for a variety of cell classification problems [115], such as classification of different types of leukocytes using microscopic images [116], cancer cells exposed to drugs based on their trajectories [117], and immune cells and tumor cells using biophysical features extracted from optical phase and loss images [118]. Recently, machine learning-based approaches have been used for T cell classification, in which quantitative variables such as autofluorescence lifetime [106], or morphological variables [105] are extracted from images and used to classify quiescent and activated T cells, or cognate and non-cognate T cell – DC contacts, respectively. However, these models are limited by the need for long T cell activation times (Table 3.1), and the model by Liarski et al. [105] in particular, omits critical temporal information that can be used to improve classification accuracy.

Here, we use deep learning to classify cognate, antigen-specific T cells by leveraging the unique interaction dynamics between cognate and non-cognate T cells-DCs observed as naive T cells scan DCs for the presence of the cognate pMHC complex in lymphoid organs [40]. Contact between T cells and cognate DCs results in changes in T cell morphology and motility, whereby T cells either immediately, or after some period of transient interactions called kinapses, flatten against the cognate DC and form stable, long-lasting interactions called synapses [33, 119]. T cells interacting with non-cognate DCs, on the other hand, scan and make transient interactions with many DCs, and do not exhibit the same changes as those making stable cognate interactions [40]. Furthermore, the activation of memory T cells following re-infection also depends predominantly on interactions with DCs [120]. Thus, many types of T cell responses are directed by DCs *in vivo*. We hypothesize that a deep learning model, aided by anti-CD40 antibodies (aCD40), can classify $CD8^+$ T cells interacting with cognate DCs, and $CD8^+$ T cells interacting with non-cognate DCs, based on their distinct interaction dynamics in terms of morphology and motility. This model could be used to rapidly identify cognate and non-cognate T cell – DC interactions to better understand their role in disease progression, and, upon integration in a cell-sorting device, could be used to simplify and enhance the enrichment and selection of antigen-specific T cells for use in ACT.

3.2 Methods

3.2.1 Mice

All animal procedures were approved by the Columbia University Institutional Animal Care and Use Committee (IACUC) and all experiments were performed in accordance with relevant guidelines/regulations. C57BL/6J (B6), C57BL/6-Tg(TcraTcrb)1100Mjb/J (OT-I), B6.Cg-Tg(TcraTcrb)425Cbn/J (OT-II), NOD/ShiLtJ (NOD), and NOD.Cg-Tg(TcraTcrbNY8.3)1Pesa/DvsJ (NY8.3) mice were purchased from The Jackson Laboratory.

3.2.2 Cell culture

JAWS II DCs were purchased from ATCC, the DO-11-10 T cell hybridoma was purchased from Sigma, and BALB/c bone marrow-derived DCs (BMDCs) were purchased from Cell Biologics. Cultured primary cells: Bone marrow cells were harvested from the tibia and femur of mice, and they were pre-enriched for DC differentiation by removing CD3+, Gr-1+ and B220+ cells using biotinylated anti-Gr-1 (RB6-8C5), biotinylated anti-CD3 (17A2) and biotinylated anti-B220 (RA3-6B2) antibodies (BioLegend) with magnetic streptavidin MACS beads (Miltenyi). The pre-enriched bone marrow cells were cultured with 20 ng/mL GM-CSF (PeproTech) for 7-10 days, and harvested from the flasks and enriched for CD11c+ BMDCs using CD11c MACS beads (Miltenyi) on the final day of culture. BMDCs were stained with a deep red cell tracker (Thermo Fisher) for 15-20 minutes in PBS. The spleen was harvested from mice (between 7 and 10 weeks of age), and CD8$^+$ T cells were purified from splenocytes using a naive CD8+ T cell isolation kit (Miltenyi), CD8$^+$ T cell isolation kit (Miltenyi), or naive CD4$^+$ T cell isolation kit (Miltenyi). T cells were stained with calcein (Thermo Fisher) for 15 minutes in full media.

3.2.3 Cell culture media

JAWS II DCs were cultured in media which was 80% Minimum Essential Medium (with Alpha Modification, ribonucleosides, deoxyribonucleosides) (Millipore Sigma) with 1% L-Glutamine (L/G) (Thermo Fisher), 1 mM sodium pyruvate (Thermo Fisher), 5 ng/ml GM-CSF (PeproTech), and 20% FBS (Thermo Fisher). The DO-11-10 T cell hybridoma was cultured in RPMI-1640 (Thermo Fisher) with 1% L/G and 10% FBS. Bone marrow cells were cultured in RPMI-1640 with 10% FBS, 1% L/G, 1% P/S (Sigma-Aldrich), 20 ng/mL GM-CSF, 50 μM beta mercaptoethanol (Thermo Fisher) and 0.1 mg/mL Normocin (Invivogen). When T cells were co-cultured with BMDCs, the cells were cultured in splenocyte media: RPMI-1640 with 10% FBS, 1% MEM non-essential amino acids (Thermo Fisher), 1% sodium pyruvate, 1% L/G, 1% P/S, 50 μM beta mercaptoethanol, 0.02 mg/mL Gentamycin (Thermo Fisher), 0.5 μg/mL Amphotericin B (Thermo Fisher).

3.2.4 Experimental setup

Purified and fluorescently labeled BMDCs were cultured on fibronectin-coated (10 μg/cm^2) 8-well chambered cover glass slides (Labtek) at a concentration of 1.6×10^5 cells per well, with 1 μg/mL LPS overnight. The next day, the BMDCs were washed, and media with the 10 μg/mL of the appropriate peptide (cognate wells), or with media alone (non-cognate wells) was added to the BMDCs. The N4 peptide OVA$_{257\text{-}264}$ (SIINFEKL) or variant Q4 peptide OVA$_{257\text{-}264}$ (SIIQFEKL) were used for OT-I experiments, the IGRP$_{206\text{-}214}$ peptide (VYLKTNVFL) was used for NY8.3 experiments, and the OVA$_{323\text{-}339}$ peptide (ISQAVHAAHAEINEAGR) was used for OT-II and DO-11-10 experiments. Note that the Q4 peptide is reported to have a 18-fold lower functional avidity [121], and a 6.5 fold lower 2D affinity [122], than the N4 peptide. After 3 hours of peptide pulsing, some wells were incubated with 10 µg/mL anti-ICAM-1 (YN1/1.7.1; Thermo Fisher) or 0.01 mg/mL anti-CD40 (HM40-3; BioLegend) antibodies for 10 minutes, and then the BMDCs were washed. Purified, calcein-labeled $CD8^+$ T cells were then added to each well at a concentration of $5x10^4$ cells per well. These cell densities were selected to ensure contact between T cells and DCs, while enabling accurate tracking of the T cells. The cells were then imaged on a Nikon spinning-disk confocal microscope using a 20x objective. The cells were maintained in a humid environment with 5% CO_2 using a Tokai Hit stage-top incubator and objective heater. Time-lapse images were taken of 3 spots per well, every 1-2.5 minutes for up to 80 minutes. Initial assessment of DO-11-10 T cell hybridoma activation involved co-culturing $2x10^4$ BMDCs with $1x10^5$ T cells in a 96 well plate (or other conditions) for 4 days, and then performing an IL-2 ELISA (R&D Systems) on the collected supernatant. To assess T cell activation for the OT-I cells, the protocol was the same, except the ratios were adjusted to more closely match the ratios of T cells to DCs used in the imaging experiments. Specifically, $1x10^5$ BMDCs were co-cultured with $5x10^4$ T cells in a 96 well plate for 3 days, at which point the supernatant was collected, and an IL-2 ELISA was performed. Note that OT-I and OT-II T cells were cultured with BMDCs harvested from C57BL/6, OT-I or OT-II mice, while NY8.3 T cells were cultured with BMDCs harvested from NY8.3 or NOD mice.

3.2.5 T cell tracking and video processing

Following image acquisition, the T cells were identified and tracked using the TrackMate plugin on Fiji [123], and the tracks were used to generate videos in the frame of reference of each individual T cell in MATLAB. A 101 px × 101 px region was cropped around the centroid at each time point in a track, and concatenated to form a video, with the T cell of interest in the middle. However, for instances where the cells were located at the edge of the original imaged region, the cell is located at the edge of the 101x101 pixel frame. All videos had at least 20 frames, and any cells with less than 20 frames were excluded. In order to ensure that only the T cell of interest was visible, any neighboring T cells were removed from each frame by using ROIs of the tracked T cell to apply a mask, which removed everything outside of the ROI, or T cell of interest. The T cells and DC channels were then blurred using the Gaussian blur filter, and then binarized. Each frame in the DC channel was binarized in Fiji using values determined by the Huang thresholding for the original image, prior to cropping, while each frame in the T cell channel was binarized using values determined by the Otsu thresholding algorithm, after cropping. A variety of thresholding methods were tested to ensure accurate and complete binarization of all T cells and DCs.

These 20-61 frame videos were used for the non-deep learning classification methods. However, classification by deep learning required all videos to have the same number of frames. As such, for the deep learning pipeline, the videos were evenly sampled to generate videos with 20 frames each. More specifically, in videos with 20-39 frames the first 20 frames were selected, in videos with 40-59 frames, every other frame was selected for a total of 20 frames, and for videos with 60-61 frames, every third frame was selected for a total of 20 frames. Videos were also generated in which either the first 20, 10, 5, or 2 consecutive frames were selected.

3.2.6 Non-deep learning quantification

After binarization, Fiji was used to determine the number of red pixels in each frame. The region of overlap between the T cell (green) and DC (red) channel was also visualized and quantified.

Based on the time between each frame, TrackMate calculated the T cell speed between each frame along a track, which was used to calculate an average speed. Circularity was also calculated in Fiji. For the preliminary experiment involving the addition of aCD40 or aICAM-1 to WT T cells and DCs, interaction time was determined by manually counting the number of frames (and thus time) each T cell remains in contact with a DC (note that all of the videos in this single experiment were sampled at the same rate, and so we could easily convert the number of frames to time). For the OT-I experiments, interaction time for each track was calculated using the overlapped data, by identifying consecutive frames in which red and green pixels were overlapping, representing the T cell interacting with a DC. Due to differences in the total time imaged for each experiment, and even for T cells within each experiment, in order to include all of the T cells, interaction time was quantified as the percentage of time each T cell interacts with a DC, during the total time imaged for that T cell.

3.2.7 Deep learning model

The deep learning model is composed of a feature extractor with 4 blocks of time distributed convolutional neural network (CNN), batch normalization and max pooling layers. The model takes in an input with the shape: (number of frames, 101 (height), 101 (width), 3 (number of channels)). The details of the feature extractor are as follows: 3x3 kernel with 8 filters (block 1 conv1), 3x3 kernel with 4 filters (block 1 conv2), batch normalization, max pooling with 2x2 pool size and 1x1 stride, 3x3 kernel with 16 filters (block 2 conv1), 3x3 kernel with 8 filters (block 2 conv2), batch normalization, max pooling with 2x2 pool size and 1x1 stride, 3x3 kernel with 32 filters (block 3 conv1), 3x3 kernel with 16 filters (block 3 conv2), batch normalization, 2x2 pool size and 1x1 stride, 3x3 kernel with 64 filters (block 4 conv1), batch normalization, 2x2 pool size and 1x1 stride. The extracted features from each frame were flattened and passed to an

long short term memory (LSTM) layer with 100 units, dropout of 0.2, recurrent dropout of 0.2,

and L2 regularizer of 0.01. Finally, the model had a fully connected layer with 100 units, and a

softmax classification layer with 2 units. The RMSprop optimizer algorithm, learning rate of 10^{-4}, and binary crossentropy loss function were used. The model was trained for 20 epochs using

80% of the videos of cognate and non-cognate OT-I T cells interacting with high affinity N4-

DCs or un-pulsed DCs, respectively (with or without aCD40), and validated using 10% of the

videos from the same groups. Training data was also randomly augmented via horizontal or

vertical shift to increase the size of the dataset. Testing was completed using 10% of the high

affinity cognate and non-cognate OT-I T cells, all of the videos of OT-I T cells interacting with

Q4-DCs, and all of the videos of NY8.3 T cells.

3.2.8 Statistical analysis

All statistical analysis was performed in GraphPad Prism 8. For pairwise comparisons, Mann-

Whitney U test was performed. For comparisons of more than 2 groups, a Kruskal-Wallis test

with Dunn's test for multiple comparisons was used. Violin plots report the median in the dashed

black line, and the quartiles in the dotted colored lines.

3.3 Results

3.3.1 Preliminary experiments to establish the model system of T cells and DCs

We initially sought to use either T cell or DC cell lines to be able to perform experiments more

rapidly. As such, we assessed whether $CD4^+$ T cells from OT-II mice could be activated by the

JAWS II DC cell line presenting the $OVA_{323-339}$ peptide, and also whether $CD4^+$ DO-11-10 T cell hybridomas could be activated by BALB/c BMDCs presenting the OVA$_{323-339}$ peptide. We assessed T cell activation by performing an IL-2 ELISA on day 3 or day 4 of co-culture, and also more qualitatively by looking for T cell cluster formation or proliferation over time. While we did not find any T cell activation by the cognate peptide-presenting JAWS II DCs, we did find activation of the DO-11-10 T cell hybridomas in response to the cognate peptide presenting BALB/c DCs. In particular, the DO-11-10 T cell hybridomas secreted IL-2 in the appropriate conditions, including with the PMA and ionomycin positive control, and with cognate peptide-presenting DCs, whereas IL-2 was not secreted in the negative controls, as expected (Fig 3.1). However, we did not move forward with using the DO-11-10 T cell hybridomas due to their rapid proliferation, even in the absence of cognate DCs, which may have interfered with or complicated the T cell tracking workflow described below. Also, T cell hybridomas have been reported to differ from naive T cells in terms of their interactions with DCs, such as by having a reduced dependence on co-stimulatory molecules [124].

Since we wanted to train a model which can be generalized to primary mouse, and eventually human, cells, for the remainder of this chapter, we mainly used primary CD8$^+$ T cells and BMDCs harvested from OT-I TCR transgenic mice, which are commonly used to study the interaction dynamics between T cells and DCs.

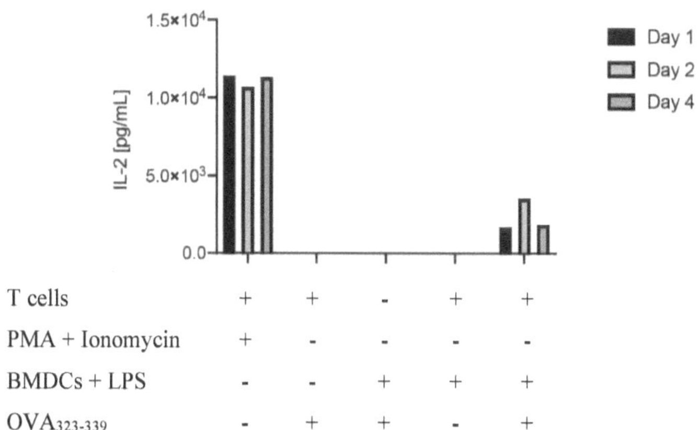

T cells	+	+	-	+	+
PMA + Ionomycin	+	-	-	-	-
BMDCs + LPS	-	-	+	+	+
$OVA_{323-339}$	-	+	+	-	+

Figure 3.1: Verification of CD4$^+$ DO-11-10 T cell hybridoma activation by BALB/c BMDCs. The supernatant was collected on day 4 of co-culture, and IL-2 secretion was quantified (n=1, mean).

3.3.2 Overview of the video processing workflow

We studied T cell – DC interactions using OT-I TCR transgenic mice, an established model system [125]. In this TCR transgenic mouse model, CD8$^+$ T cells recognize a specific peptide sequence from ovalbumin, $OVA_{257-264}$ (N4) peptide (SIINFEKL), restricted to H-2K^b MHC class I. OT-I CD8$^+$ T cells were co-cultured with N4 peptide-presenting DCs (N4-DCs) or un-pulsed DCs, and the cells were imaged every 1 to 2.5 minutes, for up to 1.5 hours (Table 3.2 for experimental details). We used an automated cell tracking software (Fig 3.2a) to track each T cell, then cropped a moving 101x101 pixel region around the centroid of the T cell, and concatenated the images to form a video in the frame of reference of the T cell. We then applied a mask to remove any neighboring T cells present in the frame to ensure that only the centered T cell of interest was visible. The T cell and DC channels were then blurred, and thresholded to remove any imaging-related or experiment-specific noise and artifacts (Fig 3.2b). Note that videos of T cells from wells consisting of T cells and N4 peptide-presenting DCs were labeled as cognate (cog) T cells, while T cells from wells consisting of T cells and un-pulsed DCs were

labeled as non-cognate (non-cog) T cells. We then used traditional image analysis techniques,

and deep learning to classify the videos of cognate and non-cognate T cells.

Table 3.2: Experimental Details

Experiment	Time between frames (min)	Max number of frames	+aCD40		-aCD40	
			Antigen-specific	Non-antigen specific	Antigen-specific	Non-antigen specific
1. OT-I	1.5	45	197 (N4)	256	195 (N4)	196
2. OT-I	2	30	-	-	227 (N4)	314
3. OT-I	2	40	179 (N4)	195	190 (N4)	174
4. OT-I	2	40	205 (Q4)	-	-	-
5. OT-II	1.5	41	219	153	178	178
6. NY8.3	1	61	94	253	109	205
7. NY8.3	1.5	46	295	304	224	227

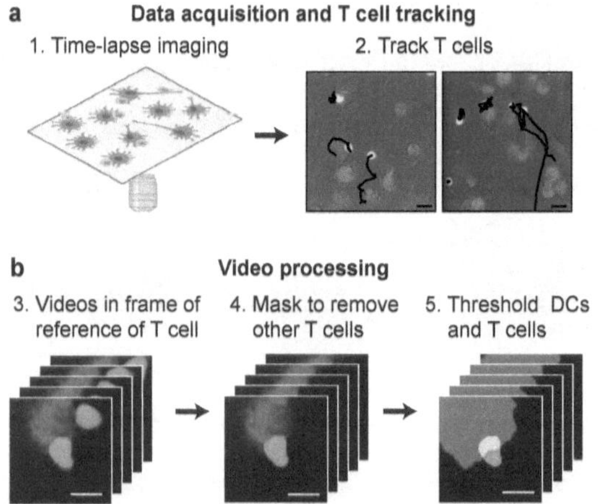

Figure 3.2: Schematic diagram of video processing. (a) Schematic of time-lapse microscopy of interacting T cells (green) and DCs (red) and subsequent automated T cell tracking (tracks in black). Scale bar is 20 μm. (b) Process to generate individual, thresholded, 101x101 pixel videos in the frame of reference of each T cell. Scale bar is 10 μm.

3.3.3 Use of anti-CD40 antibodies to improve discrimination of cognate vs. non-cognate interactions

We hypothesized that the incubation of DCs with anti-CD40 antibodies (aCD40), prior to the addition of T cells, could amplify the differences in interaction dynamics between cognate and non-cognate T cell – DCs. One possible mechanism is that CD40 agonists enable DC licensing, leading to increased expression of co-stimulatory and adhesion molecules [126] and secretion of inflammatory cytokines [127], which may reinforce cognate interactions, and improve the ability of DCs to discriminate between cognate and non-cognate T cells to also reduce non-specific binding between non-cognate T cells and DCs.

We performed a preliminary study to assess the effect of aCD40 and anti-ICAM-1 antibodies (aICAM-1) on non-cognate interactions between T cells and DCs, by culturing $CD8^+$ T cells from WT B6 mice with DCs alone or with DCs cultured with aCD40 or aICAM-1 antibodies. We found that the addition of aCD40 and aICAM-1 reduced long-term interactions between T cells and DCs (Fig 3.3a), thereby reducing non-specific interactions between non-cognate T cells and DCs (as was previously demonstrated for aICAM-1). However, here we chose to avoid blocking ICAM-1 because it has been demonstrated to also reduce long-term interactions between cognate T cell – DCs, whereas we aimed to preferentially reduce long-term contacts only between non-cognate T cells – DCs. We initially hypothesized that the aCD40-mediated reduction in long-term non-specific binding between non-cognate T cells and DCs was due to interfering between CD40-CD40L interactions between DCs and $CD8^+$ T cells, respectively (since some activated $CD8^+$ T cells express CD40L [128]), similar to how the deletion of ICAM-1 signaling in DCs reduced long-term binding with non-cognate T cells [129]. However, since the DCs are only incubated with the agonistic aCD40 antibodies for ~10 mins, it is likely that the

CD40 molecules would be recycled and presented again on the cell surface. Thus, there may be

other aCD40-mediated mechanisms which can reduce non-specific binding. To ensure that the

addition of aCD40 did not impact cognate T cell – DC interactions, or T cell activation, we

measured IL-2 secretion on day 3 of T cell – DC co-culture, and found similar levels of IL-2

between co-cultures of cognate T cell – DCs incubated with or without aCD40 (Fig 3.3b).

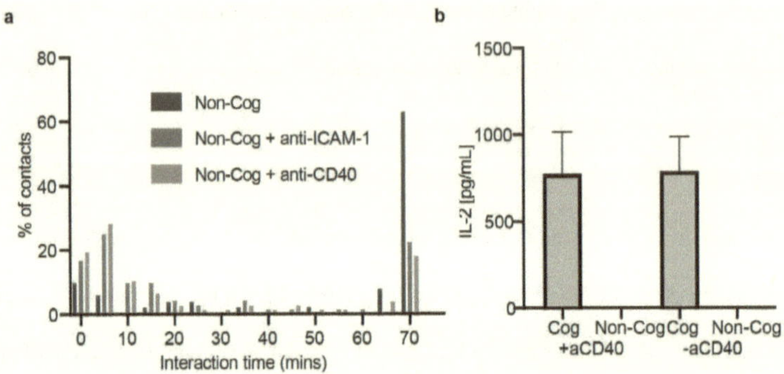

Figure 3.3: The effect of antibodies on T cell – DC interactions. (a) Non-cognate T cells and DCs were incubated alone, with anti-CD40 antibodies, or anti-ICAM-1 antibodies to determine their effect on non-specific interactions (mean, n=1). (b) Cognate and non-cognate T cell – DCs were co-cultured with or without anti-CD40 antibodies for 3 days to determine its effect on T cell activation in terms of IL-2 secretion (mean ± standard deviation, n=3).

3.3.4 Traditional image analysis methods for classification of OT-I T cell – DC interactions

We first applied traditional image analysis techniques for classifying T cell – DC interactions.

Specifically, we first quantified the total area of the T cells and DCs in each frame by

determining the total number of binarized green and red pixels, respectively (Fig 3.4). The

average number of overlapped pixels, between T cells and DCs, that are present in both the red

and green channels (Fig 3.4) was then quantified as an indicative measurement of proximity

between the two cell types. The average number of red pixels was also quantified because

cognate T cells spend more time in close proximity to DCs than non-cognate T cells. Note that the average number of red pixels in the pre-processed/un-cropped videos is the same in all of the

conditions (Fig 3.5), and so any differences in red pixels between cognate and non-cognate T

cells is not due to differences in initial DC numbers, but rather due to the greater propensity of

cognate T cells to be in contact with DCs. Speed is a common classification metric because

cognate T cells typically have lower velocities due to their longer interaction times with DCs,

while non-cognate T cells rapidly scan DCs with minimal long-term interactions [130]. As such,

we also quantified the percentage of time each T cell interacts with a DC, as an indicative

measurement of interaction time. Finally, we also used average circularity as a classification

metric in order to account for the differences in morphology between cognate and non-cognate T

cells as they interact with DCs.

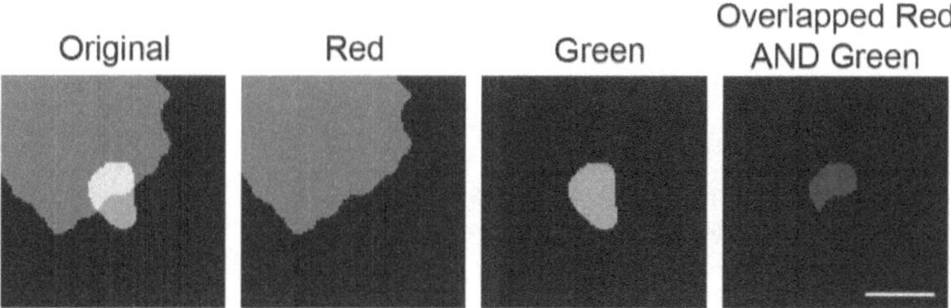

Figure 3.4: Example frame separated into individual red and green channels, as well as the region of overlap between the red and green channels. These were used to quantify red pixels, and overlapped pixels.

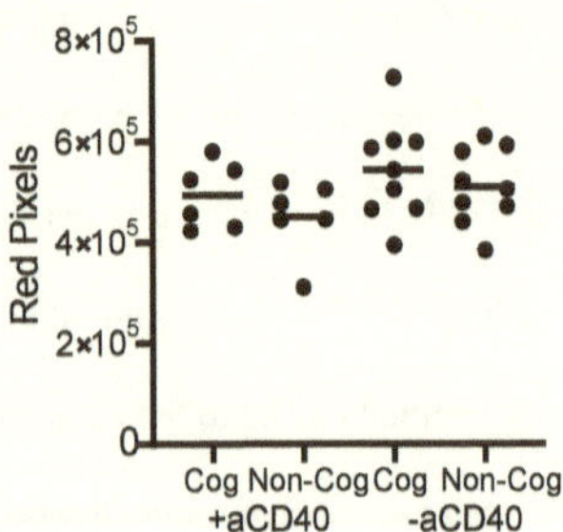

Figure 3.5: Quantification of red pixels in the original videos. The average number of red pixels over all of the frames in the original videos was calculated in order to determine whether there were differences in the number of red pixels, and thus, the number of DCs, prior to cropping into individual videos.

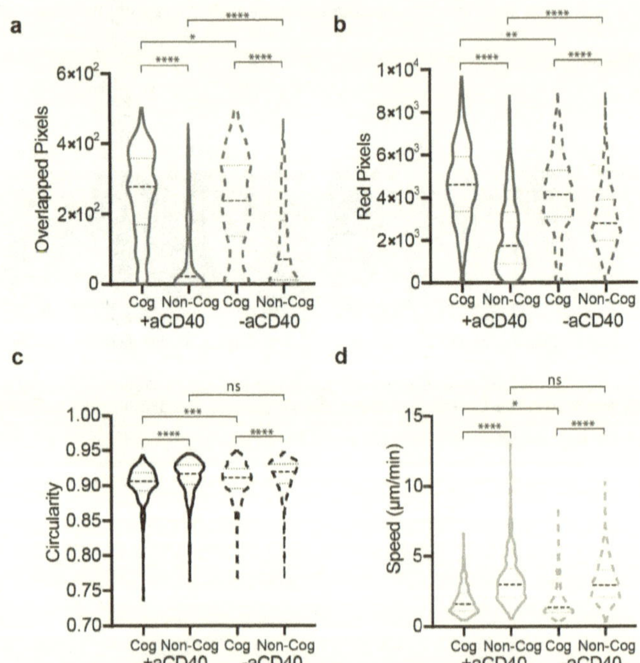

Figure 3.6. Using traditional image analysis methods to classify cognate vs. non-cognate T cell – DC interactions, with or without aCD40. (a-d) Distributions of (a) overlapped pixels (b) red pixels (c) circularity and (d) speed for cognate and non-cognate OT-I T cells incubated with or without aCD40, averaged over all of the frames in the video.

64

As expected based on what is known about the motility and morphology of cognate T cells in comparison to non-cognate T cells as they interact with DCs, there were significantly more overlapped pixels and red pixels, and significantly lower speed and circularity in cognate T cells in comparison to non-cognate T cells, both with and without anti-CD40 (Fig 3.6, 3.7). The overlapped pixel data was also used to visualize T cell interactions with DCs over time, and it can be seen that cognate T cells spend more time in contact with DCs in comparison to non-cognate T cells (Fig 3.8a-b). The degree of discrimination between cognate and non-cognate T cells for all of the parameters was quantified by the area under the curve (AUC) of a receiver-operator curve (ROC) (Table 3.3, Fig 3.7, 3.8c) which plots the true positive rate (sensitivity) vs. false positive rate (1-specificity) for a variety of cut-off values. While circularity provided a mediocre discrimination, the rest of the metrics were able to more robustly distinguish between cognate and non-cognate T cells, especially in the presence of aCD40 (summarized in Table 3.3). We found that the overlapped pixels metric, with aCD40, provided the best discrimination between cognate and non-cognate T cells, with an AUC of 0.86. This was comparable to the machine learning model developed by Liarski et al. [105], who trained a model to classify static images of T cells interacting with cognate or non-cognate DCs using extracted distance and morphology parameters, and achieved an AUC of 0.84.

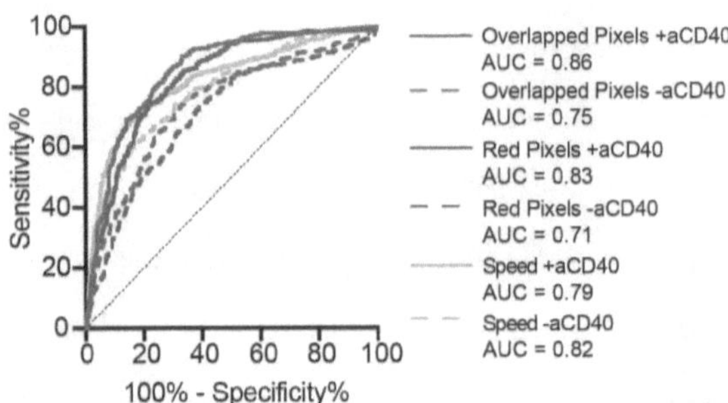

Figure 3.7. ROC quantifying the ability of the different metrics (overlapped pixels, red pixels, speed), with or without aCD40, to discriminate between cognate and non-cognate T cells.

With the exception of speed, the addition of aCD40 resulted in a higher AUC, and thus, greater

discrimination between cognate and non-cognate T cells for all of the metrics tested, in

comparison to the absence of aCD40 (Table 3.3). The addition of aCD40 served to improve the

classification by enhancing the differences between cognate and non-cognate T cells. For

example, the addition of aCD40 significantly decreased the number of overlapped pixels and red

pixels in non-cognate T cells, while it significantly increased the same metrics in cognate T cells

(Fig 3.6a-b). However, while the addition of aCD40 to non-cognate T cell – DCs did not

significantly impact T cell speed or circularity (shape), it significantly decreased the circularity

of cognate T cells (Fig 3.6c-d). Unexpectedly, we found that the addition of aCD40 significantly

increased the speed of cognate T cells, which could be attributed to changes in DC speed, since

the DCs were also motile, and thus T cell speed could not be easily decoupled from DC speed.

However, in the majority of cases, the addition of aCD40 further amplified the differences

between cognate and non-cognate T cell – DCs, which improved the classification accuracy

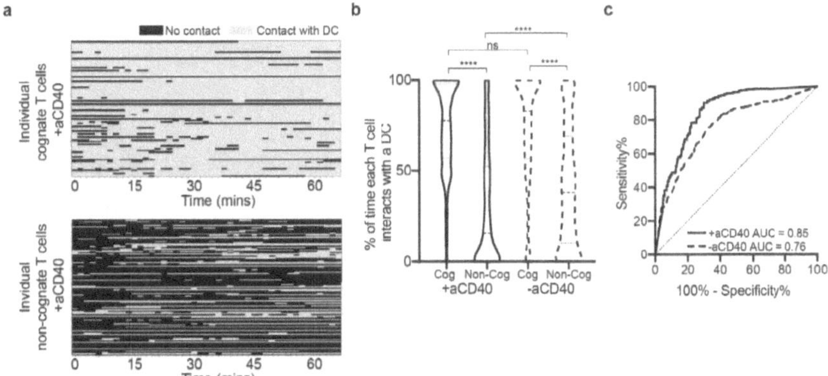

Figure 3.8. Classifying cognate and non-cognate T cells using a temporal metric. (a) Visual representation of +aCD40 cog T cell (top) and +aCD40 non-cog T cell (bottom) interactions with DCs over the course of the experiment. A subset of the T cells which were imaged for around 68 minutes are visualized. This was generated using the overlapped pixel data set, in that a T cell was considered to be interacting with a DC (yellow) if they had some degree of overlap in a frame. (b) Interaction time was quantified as a percentage of time each cog or non-cog T cell interacts with DCs, when incubated with or without aCD40. (c) ROC quantifying the ability of this temporal metric to discriminate between cognate and non-cognate T cells.

Table 3.3: Summary of OT-I T cell AUCs

	AUC	
	+aCD40	**-aCD40**
Red pixels	0.83	0.71
Overlapped pixels	0.86	0.75
% of time each T cell interacts with DCs	0.85	0.76
Speed	0.79	0.82
Circularity	0.64	0.59

3.3.5 Deep learning for classification of OT-I T cell – DC interactions

3.3.5.1 Model architecture

After establishing a baseline degree of classification using image analysis techniques, we trained

a CNN-LSTM binary classifier (Fig 3.9) to more accurately classify videos of cog or non-cog

OT-I T cells, either with or without aCD40 (referred to as +aCD40 or -aCD40, respectively). The

CNN-LSTM network consists of CNN layers for feature extraction, an LSTM model to maintain

memory of each frame, a fully connected layer, and a final classification layer. The output of the

model is the probability that the T cell in the inputted video is making cognate interactions with

DCs (in which case it is considered an antigen-specific T cell), or non-cognate interactions with

DCs. Following training, the binary classifier was tested on cog and non-cog OT-I T cell videos

(not used during training or validation), as well as videos of different types of cog and non-cog T

cells. For the CNN-LSTM network, all of the videos were required to have the same number of

frames, so in order to maximize information, each video was reduced to a total of 20 frames

which were uniformly sampled from the original video. By varying this sampling rate and the

experimentally captured frame rate, we ensured that the model could robustly classify T cells,

independently of the sampling rate.

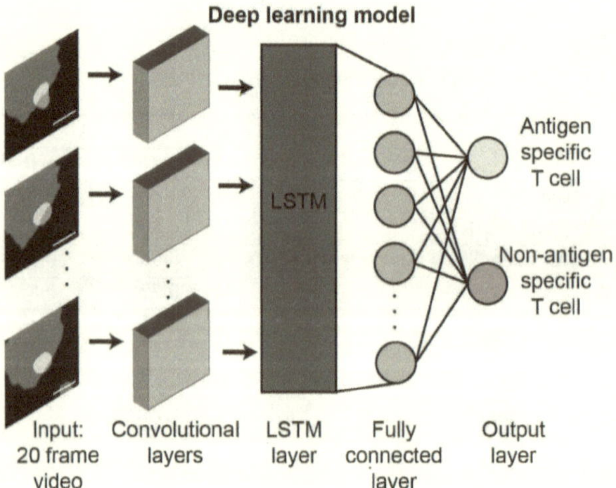

Figure 3.9: Overview of the deep learning-based binary classifier. The model consists of a feature extractor (with time distributed CNN, batch normalization and max pooling layers), LSTM model, fully connected layer, and final softmax classification layer to classify T cells as making cognate or non-cognate interactions with DCs. Scale bar is 10 μm.

3.3.5.2 Deep learning of videos processed differently resulted in overfitting

Although we ultimately used binarized videos to classify T cells, we initially tried to use non-binarized videos that included the brightfield channel. To do so, we used the model described in Fig 3.9, however, with slightly different input videos. We initially sought to include the brightfield channel because certain DC features, such as dendrites, were more clearly visible under brightfield than under fluorescence alone. We similarly assessed deep learning models which were trained on videos composed of the red and green channels alone, red channel alone, green channel alone, and the brightfield channel alone. However, any model which was trained on videos including the brightfield channel overfit the training data; it performed very well on the test data originating from the same experiment, but did not generalize well to datasets from other experiments. We hypothesized that this may have been because within one experiment, all of the videos of cognate T cells came from one well, while all of the videos of the non-cognate T cells came from another well, and so the model may have learned features specific to those wells, such as some intrinsic noise or the background intensity. To overcome this issue, we histogram matched the videos in order to normalize the grayscale intensity values across all of the frames, for all of the videos. However, even after histogram matching, the model could not generalize well to videos from different experiments. After ruling out the brightfield data, the model was then trained using videos with non-thresholded red and green channels. In this case, the model could not accurately classify videos from the same experiment (AUC = 0.8) or from different experiments. This is likely due to large fluctuations in intensity that occur across space and time, and in certain examples, the T cell and DC overlap lead to obstruction of the T cell signal. To account for this spatiotemporal variation in intensity, we applied an adaptive thresholding method to obtain a more representative image of the T cells. The adaptive thresholding process required substantial optimization, in terms of the binarizing algorithm used, whether the channels were binarized before or after cropping, and whether the same threshold was applied across all of the frames. Due to the even staining of the T cells, the thresholding process (adaptively thresholding each frame after cropping) accurately visualized the whole cell. However, due to the diffuse staining of the DC dendrites, variable amounts of the dendrites could be captured depending on the threshold selected. In order to be consistent, for each frame, we thresholded the red (DC) channel prior to cropping to ensure the DCs within the same frame were equally captured. Thus, the final video processing workflow entailed thresholding the red and green channels and removing the brightfield channel.

3.3.5.3 Deep learning results

Using the thresholded images, we were able to robustly train a model without overfitting, using data augmentation, optimizing the architecture of the model, and including regularization terms. Two separate binary classifiers were trained to distinguish cognate and non-cognate T cells using samples with or without aCD40. In each case, 80% of the videos were used for training, 10% for validation, and 10% for testing, with the +aCD40 classifier achieving training and validation accuracies around 85%, with steadily decreasing loss (Fig 3.10). Overall, the +aCD40 binary classifier provided better discrimination between cognate and non-cognate T cells (Fig 3.11a), yielding an AUC of 0.91, while the -aCD40 model yielded an AUC of 0.75 (Fig 3.11b). In line with the non-deep learning methods, the presence of aCD40 resulted in more effective classification, and as such, in the work below, we only consider the models trained and tested using samples with aCD40.

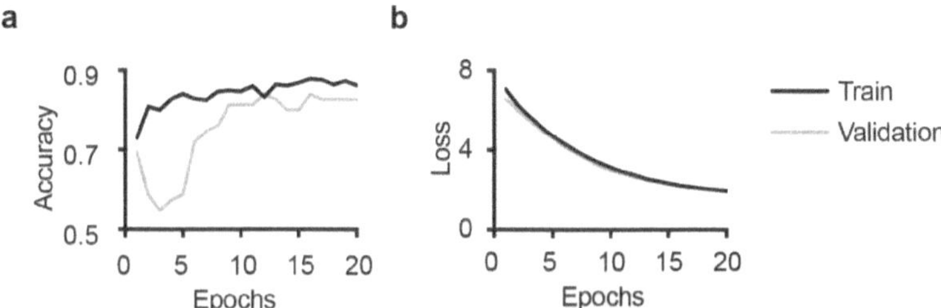

Figure 3.10: Training the +aCD40 model. (a) Accuracy curve (b) Loss curve.

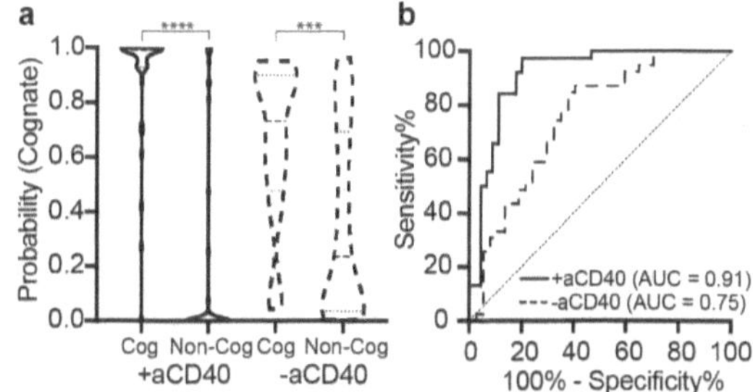

Figure 3.11: Using deep learning to classify cognate vs. non-cognate T cell – DC interactions, with or without aCD40. (a) Predicted probability that an OT-I T cell is cognate using models trained and tested on datasets with or without aCD40. (b) ROC curves quantifying the ability of the deep learning models to discriminate between cognate and non-cognate T cells based on the probabilities predicted in (a).

In order to interpret the +aCD40 model, we examined videos from the test set which were correctly predicted as being cognate (Fig 3.12a) and non-cognate (Fig 3.12b), with a high probability. Consistent with what is known about the interaction dynamics between cognate T cells and DCs, the correctly predicted cognate T cell remained in contact with the same DC for almost the entire duration of the video (Fig 3.12a), while the non-cognate T cell quickly detached from a DC after 3 frames of contact (Fig 3.12b). We also implemented Gradient-weighted Class Activation Mapping (Grad-CAMs) to visualize the regions activated by the penultimate convolution block which are important to the designated classification in red (bottom of Fig

3.12a, 3.12b, with DCs overlaid in white, and the T cell overlaid in black) [131]. According to

the Grad-CAMs, the areas of importance for cognate T cell classification was the overlapped

region between T cells and DCs, which was consistent with our previous, simple analysis. In

contrast, when identifying non-cognate T cells, the regions of importance were less consistent.

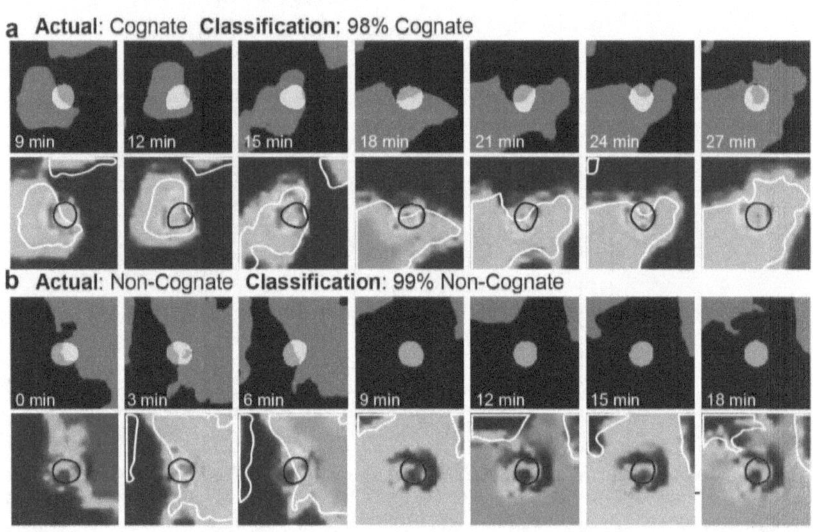

Figure 3.12: Examples of T cells which were correctly, and with a high probability classified as (a) cognate, and (b) non-cognate. The Grad-CAM heatmaps (bottom of (a) and (b)) visualize the regions important for the designated classification in red (DC outline is overlaid in white, and T cell outline is overlaid in black).

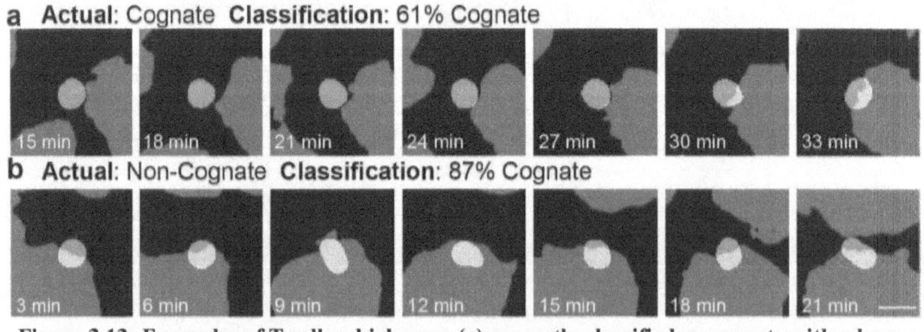

Figure 3.13: Examples of T cells which were (a) correctly classified as cognate with a lower confidence and (b) incorrectly classified as cognate. Scale bar is 10 µm.

To further probe the results of the model, we also examined examples of T cells which were correctly predicted as cognate but with a lower confidence (Fig 3.13a), and those which were incorrectly predicted as cognate but with high confidence (Fig 3.13b). The reduced predicted probability (0.61) of being cognate in Fig 3.13a may have been due to the lack of substantial overlap between the T cell and DC, despite being next to each other for at least 5 frames. The non-cognate T cell in Fig 3.13b was likely incorrectly predicted as being cognate, and with a high probability (0.87) due to the substantial overlap between the T cell and DC. The Grad-CAMs and analysis of inaccurately or incorrectly predicted videos demonstrate the importance of overlap between T cells and DCs for accurate classification. However, given that the binary classifier had a higher AUC (0.91) than classifying based on overlapped pixels alone (AUC = 0.86), the deep learning model likely incorporates other information, other than simply the number of overlapped pixels.

3.3.6 Performance of model, without adjustment of weights, to classify other types of T cell – DC interactions

We explored the performance of this method, specifically using the previously trained +aCD40 deep learning model without any adjustments in weights, for classifying other types of cognate and non-cognate T cell – DCs interactions. First, we tested the model using videos of OT-I T cells interacting with DCs pulsed with the Q4 peptide (Q4-DCs), which have a lower affinity to OT-I CD8$^+$ T cells in comparison to N4-DCs. It has been previously demonstrated that T cells interacting with Q4-DCs remained motile albeit slower, while T cells interacting with N4-DCs were arrested [130]. Consistent with previous observations, we found that T cells interacting with Q4-DCs had a mean speed in between that of T cells interacting with N4-DCs, and T cells interacting with non-cognate DCs (Fig 3.14a). Despite these differences in T cell speed, the interaction dynamics of T cells interacting with Q4-DCs were nearly indistinguishable to T cells interacting with N4-DCs in terms of overlapped pixels and red pixels (Fig 3.14b-c). By testing the binary classifier with cognate T cells interacting with Q4-DCs, we found that the model was able to accurately classify the lower affinity cognate T cells as well (Fig 3.14d).

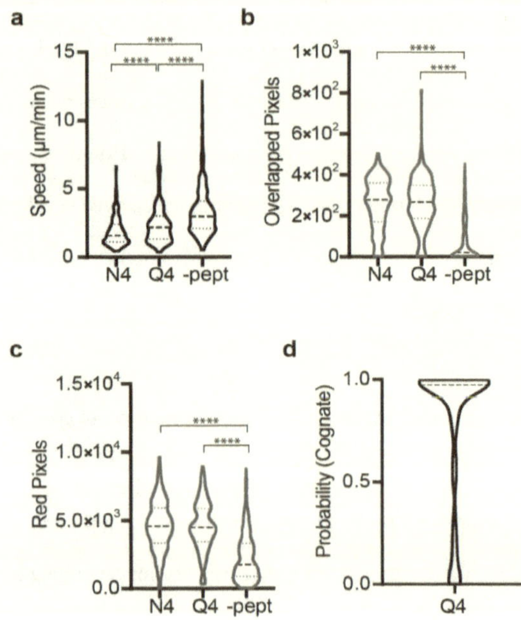

Figure 3.14: +aCD40 deep learning model trained on one set of interacting T cells and DCs accurately classifies OT-I CD8$^+$ T cells interacting with DCs presenting the lower affinity Q4 peptide. (a-c) Non-machine learning-based comparison of videos of OT-I cells interacting with cognate DCs presenting high affinity N4 peptides (N4), cognate DCs presenting low affinity Q4 peptides (Q4), or non-cognate un-pulsed DCs (-pept) in terms of average (a) T cell speed (b) overlapped pixels and (c) red pixels. (d) Testing of the +aCD40 deep learning model (previously trained on videos of OT-I T cells interacting with un-pulsed, or high affinity N4 peptide-pulsed DCs (N4-DCs)) on T cells interacting with DCs presenting the Q4 peptide.

Next, we assessed the ability of the model to be generalized to CD8⁺ T cells from a different

mouse strain. In particular, we tested the same model using CD8⁺ T cells from NY8.3 TCR

transgenic mice, which are reactive against an epitope from the pancreatic islet cell antigen islet-

specific glucose-6-phosphatase catalytic subunit related protein (IGRP) in the context of H2-K^d

MHC Class I, and are involved in the development of Type 1 diabetes in NOD mice. The

aCD40+ model was able to discriminate well between cognate and non-cognate NY8.3 T cells,

yielding an AUC of 0.87 (Fig 3.15). Furthermore, the deep learning model was able to

differentiate between cognate and non-cognate NY8.3 T cells better than the average number of

overlapped pixels (AUC = 0.79) or the average number of red pixels alone (AUC = 0.75) (Fig

3.15).

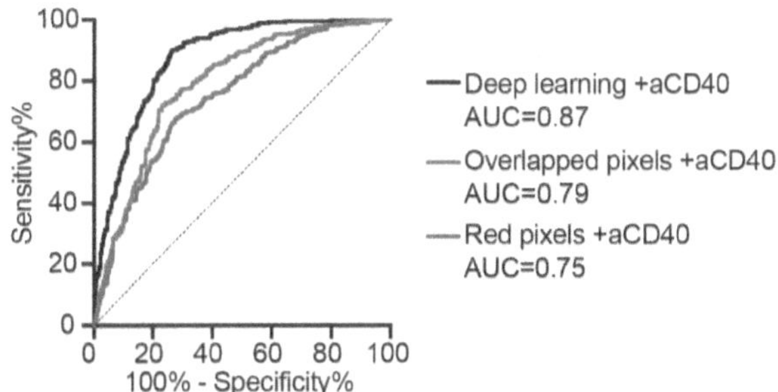

Figure 3.15: +aCD40 deep learning model trained on one set of interacting T cells and DCs accurately classifies NY8.3 CD8⁺ T cells interacting with DCs. ROC curves quantifying the ability of the +aCD40 deep learning model, overlapped pixels and red pixels to classify cognate or non-cognate NY8.3 T cells (cultured with aCD40).

Nevertheless, we observed some limitations of this method. In particular, this model (even with

+aCD40) was not able to classify CD4⁺ T cells from OT-II TCR transgenic mice (in contrast to

previously tested CD8⁺ T cells) (Fig 3.16). Speed, overlapped pixels and red pixels similarly

resulted in mediocre discrimination between cognate and non-cognate OT-II CD4⁺ T cells (Fig

3.16). This lack of generalizability to CD4⁺ T cells is likely due to differences in the interaction dynamics between CD8[+] T cells and DCs (via peptide-MHCI complexes) and CD4[+] T cells and

DCs (via peptide-MHCII complexes) [132]. Thus, a separate binary classifier likely has to be

trained using cognate and non-cognate CD4[+] T cells, in order to classify CD4[+] T cells.

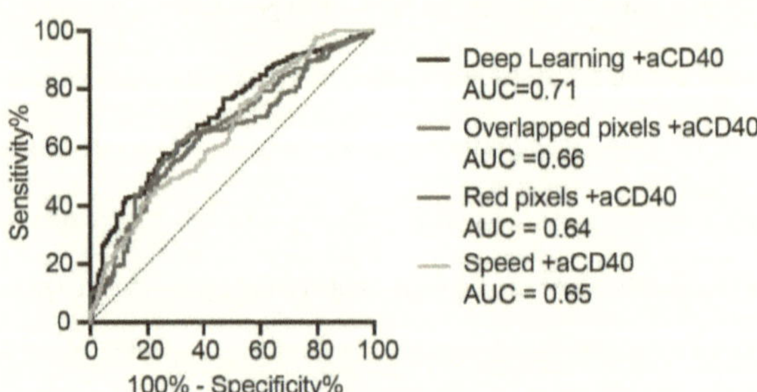

Figure 3.16: +aCD40 deep learning model trained on one set of interacting T cells and DCs does not generalize well to OT-II CD4[+] T cells. Overlapped pixels, red pixels and speed also provide mediocre discrimination between cognate and non-cognate CD4[+] T cell – DCs.

Finally, we assessed whether the deep learning model could be trained to classify shorter videos

of OT-I high affinity cognate and non-cognate T cells, and whether these models trained on

shorter videos could still be generalized to the NY8.3 CD8[+] T cells. Until this point, the deep

learning model was trained and tested using 20-frame videos which were generated by evenly

sampling the original videos, which corresponded to a time frame ranging from 20-80 minutes

(Table 3.2). We next instead trained and tested new models with videos with shorter time frames.

In particular, we generated new videos of interacting OT-I T cells and DCs consisting of 20, 10,

5 or 2 consecutive frames, where 20 consecutive frames corresponded to a time frame ranging

from 20-40 minutes. As the number of consecutive frames in the videos was decreased, the AUC

decreased as well, when tested on either the OT-I or NY8.3 T cells (Fig 3.17). Taken altogether,

this demonstrates that temporal data is necessary, and that the classification accuracy increases with more frames, and with more time. However, the models which were trained and tested using

20 consecutive frames had an AUC (0.89 for OT-I and 0.84 for NY8.3), which was comparable

to the models trained and tested using 20 evenly sampled frames (0.91 for OT-I and 0.87 for

NY8.3). Thus, the AUC does eventually plateau, and an accurate classification could be made

after up to 40 minutes of interactions, rather than up to 80 minutes.

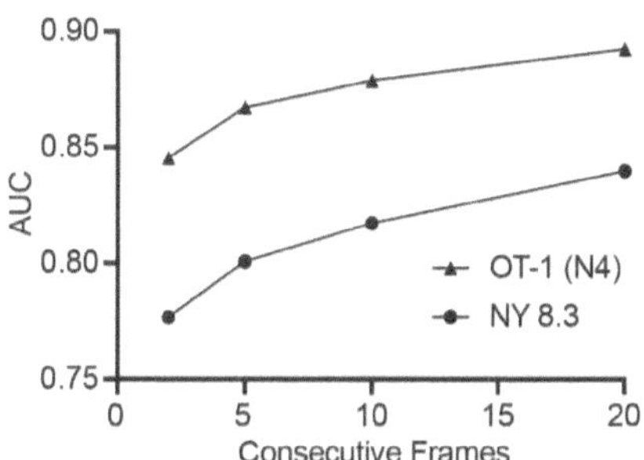

Figure 3.17: Assessment of the ability of the deep learning model to classify high affinity cognate- and non-cognate OT-I and NY8.3 T cells when trained and tested on videos of varying length. 20, 10, 5, 2 consecutive frames correspond to videos which were imaged for 20-40, 10-20, 5-10, 2-4 minutes, respectively.

3.4 Discussion

Here, we demonstrate the ability to rapidly classify videos of cognate and non-cognate CD8$^+$ T

cells based on their interactions with DCs, using simple image analysis techniques, and even

more accurately, using deep learning. We also show that incubating the DCs with aCD40 prior to

CD8$^+$ T cell – DC co-culture improved the classification accuracy. By conserving spatiotemporal

information about CD8$^+$ T cell – DC interactions, we achieved a higher AUC than other similar

methods, which used machine learning methods to instead classify static images of antigen-

specific and non-antigen-specific CD4$^+$ T cells based on their morphology and proximity to DCs

[105]. We also demonstrate the generalizability of this model, in that a model trained on OT-I

CD8[+] T cells was able to classify NY8.3 CD8[+] T cells, as well as OT-I CD8[+] T cells interacting with a lower affinity peptide. However, this model was not generalizable to CD4[+] T cells, which is likely due to differences in interaction dynamics between CD8[+] T cells and DCs and CD4[+] T cells and DCs [132].

This work demonstrated the ability to accurately classify videos of cognate and non-cognate CD8[+] T cells based on their interactions with DCs in a rapid manner. We classified T cells within approximately 20-80 minutes of T cell – DC interactions, which is substantially faster than most classification methods (Table 3.1), and is essential for high-throughput applications. Although further reducing the co-culture time would be beneficial, the imaging frequency would likely have to be increased, as the results showed that reducing the number of frames analyzed over a fixed time frame resulted in a decreased classification accuracy, while analyzing a fixed number of frames collected over different time frames resulted in comparable classification accuracies.

Our deep learning model is peptide-agnostic, since it only analyzes the interaction dynamics between T cells and DCs, and hence the overall method is not limited to pre-defined peptide sequences, unlike multimer- or artificial APC- based approaches (Table 3.1). This characteristic could be beneficial when the specific peptide sequence is unknown, such as for neoantigens, where sequencing methods are used to identify somatic mutations, but the specific peptide sequence can only be predicted using computational approaches [133]. This characteristic could also be useful if the DCs are pulsed with full antigens, or tumor cell lysates rather than peptides [134].

The study demonstrated experimental and computational improvements in methodologies that resulted in significantly improved predictions. Experimentally, the addition of aCD40 amplified the differences between cognate and non-cognate interactions and significantly improved the classification accuracy. The addition of antibodies or small molecules to strengthen certain cellular behaviors, such as increasing specific interactions, or decreasing non-specific behavior, could be applied in other cell classification problems. Computationally, we found that thresholding the red (DC) and green (T cell) channels resulted in a more generalizable model. We previously trained models using videos of non-thresholded videos, as well as videos which also included the brightfield channel, however, those models quickly overfit to the training data, and were not able to be generalized to unseen data from different experiments (data not shown). By binarizing the red and green channels and removing the brightfield channel, we removed any imaging-related or experiment-specific noise and artifacts, and the model was able to generalize well to new data.

Future work can further develop the use of this method. This model can be used to identify cognate interactions between T cells and DCs to develop a deeper understanding of their role in disease progression, immunity, and tolerance [135]. Towards translational use, the classifier could be integrated into a microfluidic cell sorter to select rare antigen-specific T cells for TCR-engineered T cell therapies. However, due to the presence of false positives, this model would likely need to be used for the expansion-free enrichment of antigen-specific T cells, which could then be followed by conventional selection assays. To assess the ability of the deep learning model to enrich for antigen-specific T cells, we can further analyze the probability distributions, and resulting ROC curves (Fig 13.11) by considering different cut-off values to balance sensitivity with specificity. For example, choosing a cut-off value close to 0 (probability that a T cell is cognate) would result in a high sensitivity, but a low specificity, resulting in the selection of a large number of false positives (non-cognate T cells). To optimize for the enrichment of cognate T cells, we consider a cut-off value which maximizes the positive likelihood ratio, which represents the likelihood that a cognate T cell would be considered cognate, compared to the likelihood that a non-cognate T cell would also be considered cognate. Here, for the OT-I T cells, we achieve a maximum likelihood ratio of 11.25 at a cut-off probability of 0.9915 (sensitivity 50%, specificity 95%), which ultimately means we can enrich antigen-specific T cells by approximately 11.25 times. This means that for 1 antigen-specific T cells in 100,000 total T cells, using this method, we could enrich the antigen-specific T cells to a ratio of 1 antigen-specific T cell in ~9,000 background T cells, which would be sufficient for subsequent selection using conventional methods such as intracellular cytokine staining [57]. Thus, by integrating this model with a device which would enable T cell selection, T cells can potentially be enriched in an expansion-free manner, to quantities detectable by conventional selection methods.

Chapter 4: Microfluidic artificial lymph node to select antigen-specific T cells

4.1 Background

The selection of antigen-specific T cells from the vast T cell repertoire is an imperative step in the manufacturing of TCR-engineered T cell therapies. However, unlike the incredibly efficient lymph node (LN), which has evolved to enable the selection and activation of T cells that recognize specific foreign antigens of interest among an array of possibilities for epitopes, current T cell selection devices and assays are not able to select all antigen-specific T cells, thereby likely reducing the therapeutic efficacy [56]. Fundamental issues that complicate the *in vitro* T cell selection process are the potentially large number of antigens that T cells need to be selected against, and the extremely vast TCR repertoire in humans, of which only a few are specific for a given antigen. To address these issues large numbers of T cells must be screened, and each T cell should be screened against multiple antigens (ultimately enabling the testing of N T cells to M antigens; N to M).

A number of different *in vitro* methods exist which aim to select T cells specific to a given set of antigens; however, these methods are currently limited by their throughput or ability to scan many antigens (Table 4.1). One class of examples which enable cell-cell contact include optical tweezers or dielectrophoresis arrays, which are effective at probing the interactions between single pairs of cells, but are very limited in throughput, and can only assess one T cell to one antigen at any given time (1 to 1) [136]. Conventional bulk assays (e.g. ELISpot or intracellular cytokine staining) and microfluidic methods which enable the pairwise confinement of one T cell and one DC in arrays (microwells [137], microdroplets [103] and microfluidic cell traps [138]), improve throughput, by assessing many T cells against one antigen (N to 1) [136], but can be limited in their ability to recover live cells, and importantly, are unable to also ensure each T cell is tested against many antigens. To overcome this limitation, multiple antigens can be introduced, but in these assays, each individual T cell is still only assayed against a single antigen. For example, in bulk assays, T cells can be split into a set of subpopulations where each subpopulation is assessed against a single antigen, however, the likelihood of a rare T cell interacting with its cognate antigen-bearing DC is reduced, which is exacerbated as more antigens are assayed. As stated by Klinger et al., "A major limitation [of current techniques] is that only one antigen can be assessed at a time. To assess several antigens the sample has to be split into different aliquots. Since many antigen-specific responses involve relatively low frequency T cells and the amount of sample available is finite there are limits to the number of antigens that can be assessed. An approach enabling assessment of numerous antigens simultaneously would overcome these limitations in addition to reducing effort and cost." [139]. Given the rarity of tumor antigen-specific T cells in the TCR repertoire, it would be much more prudent to systematically assay a number of T cells, such that each T cell is assessed against all of the identified patient-specific tumor antigens (N to M), in order to have a higher chance of selecting T cells reactive to the antigens of interest. This was also recently advocated by Arnaud et al. [136] who stated that "high-throughput screening of libraries of T cells against libraries of agnostic (unbiased) APCs in miniaturized assays" is required to accurately screen for rare neoantigen-specific T cells.

A few specialized bulk assays have been developed, which can assess a variety of T cells against a library of antigens (such that each individual T cell is assessed against multiple antigens), however, they tend to be limited by their increased manufacturing burden (Table 4.1) [56, 102, 110, 140]. For example, Yossef et al. developed an improved bulk assay in which enriched tumor infiltrating lymphocytes (TILs) were clonally/oligoclonally expanded and split up such that each aliquot was co-cultured with a particular peptide pool. Although this method demonstrated improved selection of neoantigen-specific T cells in comparison to conventional TIL-screening methods, it required time-consuming (3-4 weeks), and population-distorting T cell clonal expansion [56]. MHC multimers are another type of bulk assay which can assess multiple T cells for reactivity against multiple antigens. However, conventional MHC multimers can be limited by the need for time-consuming *in vitro* enrichment prior to selection [102] (the issues associated with enrichment are further discussed in section 3.1), require the manufacturing of MHC multimers for each human leukocyte antigen (HLA) type, and require the validation of peptide binding to each specific HLA molecule [141]. Other limitations of MHC multimers include the need for predefined peptide targets which are not always available, and the inefficient selection of low affinity targets [141]. Another issue preventing current methods from selecting all antigen-specific T cells is the inability to screen large quantities of T cells (Table 4.1).

In contrast to *in vitro* methods, the *in vivo* selection of antigen-specific T cells within the T cell zone of the lymph node is extremely efficient and can select rare antigen-specific T cells without the aforementioned limitations. The structure and organization of the densely-packed T cell zone, which acts as a meeting place where sessile networks of antigen-bearing DCs scan migrating T cells to initiate T cell priming and activation, enabling the efficient screening and selection of antigen-specific T cells. Specifically, DCs are bound to and spread out along the fibroblastic reticular network (FRN), while T cells move in between and along the FRN to randomly encounter and probe the attached antigen-presenting DCs [142, 143]. This "guided random" motility strategy allows T cells to interact with many different antigen-presenting DCs, while balancing the need to remain in a location for long enough for the T cell to receive activating signals from the DCs [144]. Also, the dense nature of the LN further enables the high-throughput and efficient screening of T cells *in vivo*, as it has been estimated that 500 [145] to 5000 [99] T cells interact with each DC every hour.

Table 4.1: Other methods used to select antigen-specific T cells

Reference	Experimental setup	Screening Ratio (T cells to antigens)	Manufacturing limitations	Throughput	Interaction mechanism
[103, 146]	Pairwise microfluidic methods	N to 1	N/A	+ (10,000s per device)	Pairwise interaction with 1 T cell and 1 DC
[101]	Bulk – intracellular cytokine staining	N to 1	Enrichment before screening	++ (100,000 per well)	T cells interact with DCs under static conditions
[102]	Bulk - MHC multimers	N to M	Enrichment before screening, manufacturing of patient-specific MHC for multimer	+ (10,000s per well)	T cells interact with pMHCs on multimers
[56]	Specialized bulk	N to M	Requires clonal/oligo-clonal expansion	- (64-200 per 96-well plate)	T cells interact with DCs under static conditions
[104]	Flow-through serpentine channel	Theoretically N to M	Manufacturing of any patient-specific HLA for artificial APCs (aAPCs)	+ (1,000s per device)	Migrating T cells interact with sessile network of aAPCs
Proposed device	Bulk – Flow through microfluidic compartments	N to M	N/A	++ (1,000,000s per device)	Flowing T cells interact with sessile network of DCs

Inspired by the unique characteristics of lymph nodes, here, we developed a "microfluidic artificial LN" via directed flow through a dense antigen-presentation network, to select for antigen-specific T cells. We aimed to design a flow-through microfluidic device which recapitulates 3 characteristics of the LN that enable the efficient selection *in vivo*: 1. Structural organization of the LN that facilitates T cell – DC interactions 2. Screening of large quantities of T cells in a high-throughput manner and 3. Interactions between each T cell and multiple antigens. To achieve this, our proposed microfluidic device consists of multiple compartments, each containing microcarrier beads (MCs) coated with DCs presenting a distinct antigen. T cells are flowed unidirectionally through each compartment and by leveraging the interaction dynamics discussed in Chapters 1 and 3, the T cells are captured in the appropriate antigen-specific compartment. By using a flow-through device where T cells are sequentially assayed against each antigen, large numbers of T cells can be assayed against multiple antigens. Using a combination of analytical methods and computational simulations, we first demonstrate that this device can assay millions of T cells, each one against multiple antigens, resulting in the stable binding of antigen-specific T cells to their cognate DC within the appropriate compartment. We then experimentally demonstrate the ability to preferentially enrich for antigen-specific T cells rather than non-specific T cells within a one-compartment device, while building towards a multi-compartment device.

4.2 Methods

4.2.1 Setting up the computational fluid dynamics – agent based-model (CFD-ABM)

To computationally simulate T cell selection in our proposed microfluidic device, we developed a coupled CFD-ABM model. The first step in developing the model involved designing a mock-up of the one-compartment device (0.36 mm depth x 0.7 mm width x 1.5 mm length) in SolidWorks. We then simulated packed MCs by using a motion study to "pack" 0.15 mm diameter spheres (representative of the MCs) into the compartment. Upon exporting this mock-up into COMSOL, fluid-flow through the device was analyzed by imposing a flow rate of 0.002 µL/min at the inlet (corresponding to an average interstitial speed of 15 µm/min, which is the average speed of T cells in the lymph node), and a pressure of 0 at the outlet. Furthermore, no slip boundary conditions were imposed on all solid boundaries, and the fluid was set to have a dynamic viscosity of 0.78×10^{-2} (dyn*s)/cm (corresponding to that of cell culture medium at 37°C [147]). The steady-state Navier-Stokes equations were solved and the resulting velocity fields were exported to MATLAB, where the ABM was developed. To do so, the surface of each MC was populated with a total of 65 DCs, which all presented the same antigen. We assumed that the DCs remained completely stationary on the MCs and to simplify the analysis, we ignored the volume of the DCs and treated them as point particles. However, the DCs were modelled as having a hemispherical sphere of influence with a (dendrite to dendrite) diameter of 45 µm [148].

To computationally simulate the experimental conditions, antigen-specific, or non-antigen-specific T cells (modeled as spheres with a diameter of 10 µm) were introduced at random locations at the inlet, and T cells were advected through the device using the velocity field data imported from COMSOL. The velocity field was solved on a finite set of nodes in COMSOL, so interpolation was used to determine the velocity field at points between nodes. For the first 60 minutes, we simulated injecting T cells into the device at a density of 1×10^{6} T cells/mL, which, for the dimensions and flow rates selected in this simulated device, corresponded to two cells per minute, one of which was an antigen-specific T cell, and one of which was a non-antigen specific T cell (which could be imposed computationally). Subsequently, in order to ensure that all of the non-interacting T cells flowed to the end of the chip, for the following 90 minutes, no new T cells were injected, and only fluid was flowed through (at the same flow rate). Since this is an

ABM, we then applied rules to the agents, which were the antigen-specific T cells and DCs, to govern their interaction dynamics at each time step. Note that, the timestep was 0.0083 minutes and that we do not consider the coupling of the fluid flow to the T cells and DCs.

4.2.2 ABM rules for T cell – DC interactions

To model the interactions of the T cells and DCs, two different interaction models were used.

Simple stopping model: If at any timestep, an antigen-specific T cell was close (less than 27.5 μm, corresponding to the T cell-to-DC interaction distance) to its cognate DC, and the T cell approached the DC at a suitably slow velocity (less than 15 μm/min), the T cell would transition to making stable interactions with the cognate DC (in which case the velocity of the T cell was set to 0 μm/min).

Signal integration model: For every timestep that an antigen-specific T cell was close (less than 27.5 μm) to its cognate DC, it received some amount of signal (ranging from 0.35 to 1 depending on the TCR-pMHC affinity). This signal was integrated over time and beyond a stimulation threshold of 5, the T cell would transition to stably binding to the cognate DC. These values were selected based on Moreau et al. [149], who fit signal and threshold values to experimental data. The signal received during each interaction was normalized to the timestep, to account for differences in the timestep, such that for a larger time step, the amount of signal received would be higher than for a smaller time step.

4.2.3 Mice

All animal procedures were approved by the Columbia University Institutional Animal Care and Use Committee (IACUC) and all experiments were performed in accordance with relevant guidelines/regulations. C57BL/6J (B6), C57BL/6-Tg(TcraTcrb)1100Mjb/J (OT-I) were purchased from The Jackson Laboratory (Bar Harbor, Maine).

4.2.4 Cell culture

BMDCs and naive $CD8^+$ T cells were harvested from WT and/or OT-I mice, and cultured as described in sections 3.2.2 and 3.2.3. For these experiments, the BMDCs were either un-pulsed or pulsed with the N4 peptide.

4.2.5 Microfluidic device fabrication

Polymethyl methacrylate (PMMA) device fabrication: The PMMA components (McMaster-Carr) were designed in SolidWorks, and fabricated using a laser cutter (Universal Laser Systems) and CNC mill (Haas). Following fabrication of the PMMA components, they were soaked overnight in water and detergent, followed by sonication for 10 minutes in diH_2O, and then dried under a nitrogen stream. Assembly was as follows: the circular cell strainer (2.5 mm diameter, 75 um mesh size, Corning) was placed in its designated spot by the outlet on the top PMMA piece, a 2.5mm diameter micro O-ring (Apple Rubber) was placed around it to ensure a proper seal, an adhesive tape was aligned on the top PMMA piece, and the two (top and bottom) PMMA pieces were sandwiched together. The device was assembled under a stereoscope by using a 3D printed aligner to accurately align each of the components

Polydimethylsiloxane (PDMS) device fabrication: Device molds were designed in SolidWorks and 3D printed on a Stratasys Objet 30 Pro or Asiga MAX X35 printer. After thorough washing and UV crosslinking of the molds, they were cast with PDMS (Dow Sylgard 184; 1:8 crosslinker:base) and crosslinked at 70°C overnight. The next day the PDMS was peeled out of the mold, 1.25mm holes were punched in the inlet and outlet channels using a biopsy punch, the PDMS was cleaned using Scotch tape, and bonded to cleaned glass slides using plasma bonding. Bonding was completed by heating the microfluidic devices to 95°C for 5-10 minutes.

4.2.6 2D T cell detachment under flow

We first studied the effect of external flow on differentiating between static cognate and non-cognate T cells, using a 2D microfluidic device, in which T cells interacted with a monolayer of DCs, followed by an assessment of T cell detachment due to increasing flow rates. The microfluidic device was a single channel with one inlet and one outlet with the dimensions 0.4 mm height x 1.4 mm width x 11 mm length, and was fabricated as described above. In order to prevent bubble formation when the device was placed in the incubator, it was treated as in [150]. Briefly, immediately after bonding, the devices were flushed with 100% ethanol and immersed in a dish with 100% ethanol for 10 minutes, the dish was then placed in a vacuum desiccator for 30 minutes, the ethanol was then replaced with distilled water and placed in the desiccator for 30 more minutes, and then autoclaved. After autoclaving, the device was placed in the BSC and flushed with sterile PBS (using sterile tubing, syringes and needles) using a syringe pump, coated with fibronectin (10 μg/cm^2) for 1 hour, and washed with PBS, all of which were injected into the device at a flow rate 50 μL/min. CD11c$^+$, fluorescently labeled OT-I or B6 BMDCs were flowed into the chip at a concentration of 5×10^6 cells/mL with LPS (1 µg/mL) at a flow rate of

90 µL/min, and the device was incubated under static conditions overnight to enable DC

attachment. The next day, the devices were washed with media and then injected with either the

peptides (10 µg/mL) or media at a flow rate of 30 µL/min, and then incubated under static

conditions for 3 hours. The devices were then washed with media, and calcein-labeled naive OT-

I $CD8^+$ T cells were flowed into the device at a concentration of 5×10^6 cells/mL, and then

incubated under static conditions for 1-2 hours. Finally, the devices were moved to a Leica

DMI6000B microscope, where we performed time-lapse imaging as media was flowed through

the device at 0 µL/min (initial static conditions), 2 µL/min, 20 µL/min and 200 µL/min. The

following chips were assessed: N4-peptide presenting BMDCs with T cells, un-pulsed BMDCs

with T cells, and T cells alone (on fibronectin coated surface). Quantification involved manually

counting the number of T cells present at the initial 0 hr time point, and in the same region of

interest for sequentially higher flow rates. T cells remaining were calculated as a fraction of the

T cells at the 0 hr time point.

4.2.7 Microcarrier beads (MCs)

Sterile, uncoated MCs (Corning) were resuspended in sterile distilled water, while Cytodex 3

MCs (Cytiva) were resuspended in PBS and autoclaved for sterility. The MCs were then washed

twice in PBS, and either used as is (uncoated), or coated with fibronectin (10 µg/cm^2) on a 3D

shaker for one hour at room temperature. The MCs were then washed in PBS, resuspended in

media at a concentration of ~1000 MCs/mL and 50 µL of the solution was pipetted into 1 well of

a 96-well low adhesion plate (Thermo Fisher) with 2×10^5 to 3×10^5 fluorescently-labeled BMDCs

and LPS (1 µg/mL), which was incubated overnight on a 2D shaker at approximately 30 rpm.

The following day (day 1), the MCs were washed in media, and then imaged on a Nikon spinning-disk confocal microscope using a 10x or 20x objective.

4.2.8 Setup of integrated device

Preparation of the integrated microfluidic device involved bonding the device, and then sequentially flushing it with 100% ethanol, water and PBS. Calcein-labeled naive CD8$^+$ T cells from OT-I mice were resuspended in a 0.5-1% high viscosity methyl cellulose solution at a final concentration of 3×10^6 cells/mL and loaded into a 1mL syringe (BD) or 0.5 mL syringe (Hamilton). Alternatively, green calcein-labeled naive CD8$^+$ T cells from OT-I mice, and red calcein-labeled naive CD8$^+$ T cells from B6 mice were resuspended in a 0.5-1% high viscosity methyl cellulose solution at a 1:1 ratio, and at a final concentration of 3×10^6 cells/mL, and loaded into a syringe. Simultaneously, the N4-DC-coated MCs from 1-2 were resuspended in 0.5 mL of 0.5-1% high viscosity methyl cellulose solution and loaded into a 1mL syringe. In order to successfully run the experiment without any backflow as the flow was switched from injecting the DC-coated MCs to injecting the T cells, the following steps were required: 1. The syringes with T cells and DCs were both connected to the microfluidic device 2. The DC-coated MCs were injected into the chip at a flow rate of 30 µL/min (the clamp on the tubing connected to the DC-coated MCs syringe was opened, while the clamp on the tubing connected to the T cell syringe was closed) 3. The syringe pump controlling the T cell syringe was turned on at a flow rate of 1 µL/min 4. The clamp on the tubing connected to the T cell syringe was opened 5. Immediately after, the clamp on the tubing connected to the DC-coated MCs syringe was closed, and the corresponding syringe pump was turned off and 6. The flow rate of the T cells was then reduced to 0.2-0.5 µL/min. Throughout all of these steps, we performed time-lapse imaging using a Leica DMI6000B microscope.

To automate the quantification of the selection of cognate T cells (labeled with green calcein) vs. non-cognate T cells (labeled with red calcein) within the device, we first thresholded each T cell channel. In order to quantify the number of attached T cells at a given time point, we had to decouple stationary cells from moving or flowing cells. As such, for each channel, the pixels (from cells) which were present in two consecutive frames were considered to be stationary, and a new image was created, consisting only of those stationary pixels. We then performed a Particle Analysis on Fiji to quantify the number stationary cells between two consecutive frames. Note that for some microfluidic devices, we imaged a few different z locations; in these cases, this analysis was performed for each z location, and the number of stationary cells between all of the layers in one device were averaged.

4.3 Results

4.3.1 Overview of the device

In order to systematically test one T cell against multiple antigens, we designed a flow-through microfluidic device consisting of a series of micro-compartments, where each compartment contains a network of packed DC-coated microcarrier (MC) beads presenting one distinct antigen. T cells can then be flowed systematically through all of the compartments, where they move through the interstitial space between MC beads and interact with antigen-presenting DCs (Fig 4.1). Importantly, as T cells pass through all of the compartments, they encounter different antigens. Based on the interaction dynamics observed to occur between T cells and DCs *in vivo*

[40] and *in vitro* [147], we anticipated that one of the following three scenarios would occur as T cells flowed through the device: (1) T cell encountering non-cognate antigen-bearing DC will scan, but not stably bind to DCs, (2) T cell encountering low affinity cognate DC will initially interact transiently and eventually stably arrest on the cognate DC, and (3) T cell encountering high affinity cognate DC will very rapidly arrest upon contacting the cognate DC. As such, antigen-specific T cells would be enriched within this device, because the T cells that remain stably bound within the compartments are specific to the antigen presented by DCs in that compartment. Finally, the stably-bound, antigen-specific T cells could be unbound and collected from each individual compartment by imposing a strong shear stress ($\sim$12 dyn/cm^2 [147]) in the transverse direction.

Fig 4.1 shows a schematic of a 3 x 1 (3 antigens/compartments x 1 parallel channel) microfluidic device in which T cells are flowed through one horizontal channel with 3 compartments, each filled with MCs coated with DCs presenting a given antigen (various versions of the actual devices are shown in Fig 4.13). Theoretically, the number of compartments can be readily scaled up to test T cells against more antigens. Also, the number of parallel channels can also be scaled up, to increase throughput and screen more T cells in a given amount of time. The workflow of the device is as follows: 1. Loading DC-antigen-coated MCs: Each compartment is isolated by closing the valves in the horizontal channel, and opening the valves in the vertical channels. DC-coated MC beads presenting one distinct antigen are flowed and packed into each compartment. 2. Flowing T cells: The valves in the horizontal valves are then opened, valves in the vertical columns are closed, and T cells are then flowed through the compartments, encountering different antigens along the way. Antigen-specific T cells will remain stably bound to its cognate

DC and the cells remaining within each compartment at the end of 24 hours are only those

specific to the antigen presented in that compartment. 3. Collection of antigen-specific T cells:

Each compartment is again isolated. Media is then flowed through each column at an increased

flow rate (2, 20, 200 µL/min, corresponding to shear stresses of 0.01, 0.1, 1 dyn/cm^2,

respectively) in order to detach and independently collect antigen-specific T cells from each

compartment.

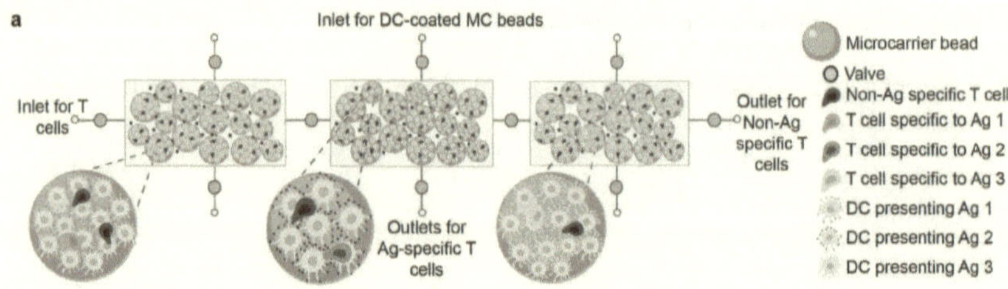

Figure 4.1: Schematic diagram of microfluidic T cell zone of lymph node. Schematic diagram of 3 antigen/compartment x 1 parallel channel (3 x 1) microfluidic device. Each compartment contains DC-coated microcarrier beads presenting one antigen. T cells are then flown through the device; T cells specific to the antigen-presenting DC in a particular compartment will remain within the compartment, while non-cognate T cells will flow through the device.

4.3.2 Feasibility analysis

Since the device was designed to assess a mixed population of T cells against a library of

antigens, we first consider whether, for given device dimensions, if it is possible to screen N T

cells against M antigens in a given amount of time t. The total number of T cells which can be

flowed through a device composed of a single parallel channel is given by:

$$N_1 = v_{int} A \phi \rho (t - \frac{LM}{v_{int}})$$
4.1

where v_{int} is the interstitial velocity of flowing T cells [µm/hr], A is the cross-sectional area of

each compartment [µm^2], ϕ is the porosity within each compartment, ρ is the injected T cell

density [cells/ µm^3], t is the time that cells are injected for [hr], L is the length of each compartment [μm], and G is the number of antigens (or compartments). Equation 4.1 quantifies

the number of T cells that accumulate at the outlet of one channel within t hours. Given a target

number of T cells N_{tot}, the number of parallel channels required is given by:

$$Number\ of\ parallel\ channels = \frac{N_{tot}}{N_1} \qquad 4.2$$

Fig 4.2 plots the number of parallel channels required to screen 10 million T cells against 30

antigens (30 compartments) in 24 hours as a function of the cross-sectional area and length of

each compartment, given the following parameters: T cell interstitial velocity of 15 μm/min (as

is the case *in vivo*), T cell density of 10 million cells/mL, porosity of 0.36 (random close packing

of spheres), and time of 24 hours. We selected a maximum time of 24 hours, since T cells which

come in contact with their cognate DC initiate proliferation after around 24 hours, which would

complicate the assay. For a compartment cross-sectional area of 10 mm^2, and a compartment

length of 400 μm, the number of parallel channels required is 29, which is a degree of

parallelization readily achieved with microfluidics.

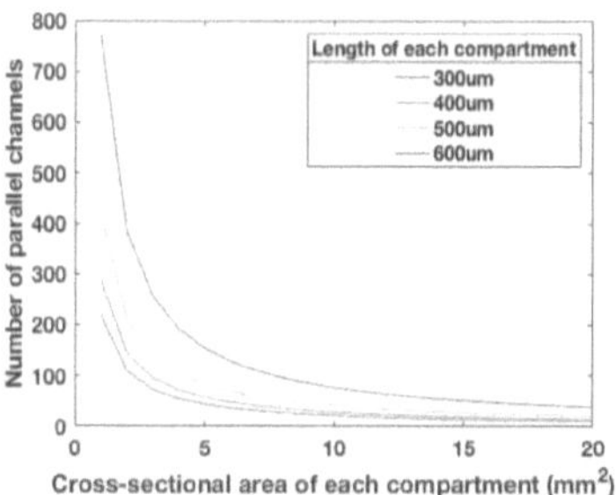

Figure 4.2: Number of parallel channels required to screen 10x10^6 T cells, as a function of compartment dimensions.

Since we have established that this device can potentially be scaled up to screen large numbers of T cells, against many antigens, in the remainder of this chapter, we focus on a one-compartment device in order to optimize various parameters, both computationally and experimentally.

4.3.3 Computational simulations: Coupled CFD – agent-based model (CFD-ABM)

To further probe the feasibility of such a device, we next developed a coupled computational fluid dynamics agent-based *in silico* model. In doing so, we aimed to quantify the ability of this type of device to efficiently select antigen-specific T cells, as well as advise device design and further probe similarities between the device and the native lymph node. Briefly, the device was designed in SolidWorks, and the velocity profile of media through the device was simulated using COMSOL Multiphysics (Fig 4.3a). The velocity data was exported to MATLAB where it was used to advect T cells in the ABM. To setup the ABM, MCs were randomly populated with DCs (Fig 4.3b,c) then T cells were introduced at the inlet and advected using the calculated velocity field, simulating the transport of T cells through the device (Fig 4.3d). In order to use this model to simulate the selection of antigen-specific T cells, we applied a set of interaction rules between T cells and DCs that governed the transition from transient to stable interactions. Those antigen-specific T cells which made stable interactions would then remain trapped within the device, while non-antigen specific ones would move to the outlet.

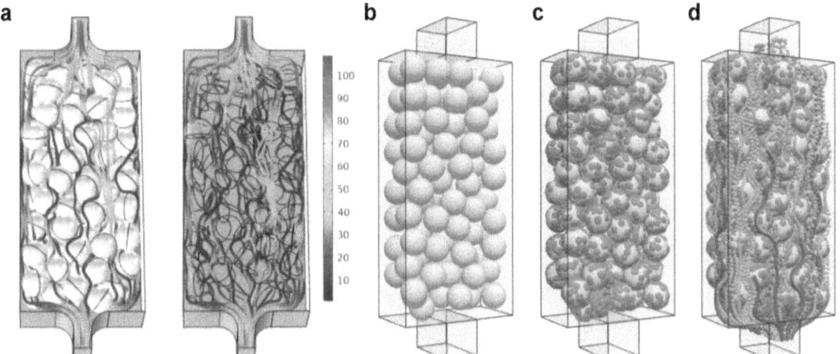

Figure 4.3: Schematic diagrams of the coupled CFD-ABM model. (a) Sample flow lines (colored by the magnitude of the velocity (μm/min)) through the device (inlet on the bottom, outlet on the top) with opaque MCs (left) and transparent MCs (right) to show that the fluid flows in the interstitial spaces. (b-d) Setting up the ABM by (b) visualizing the MCs (light gray), (c) populating the MCs with DCs (dark gray), (d) introducing antigen-specific T cells (red) and non-antigen-specific T cells (green) at the inlet, and applying rules on them as they flow through the device and interact with DCs.

We implemented two different interaction rules: 1. Simple stopping model 2. T cell signal integration model where T cells integrate signals received during transient interactions, after which they transition to stable interactions upon reaching some threshold level [149].

4.3.3.1 Model 1 – Simple stopping model

In the simple stopping model, we assumed that a cognate T cell would bind to its cognate DC if they were within each other's sphere of influence (a center-to-center distance <27.5 μm) and if it approached the DC at suitably low velocity (<15 μm/min corresponding to the average speed a T cell moves in the LN). Using this simple set of rules, we found that only 84.7 ± 2.5% of antigen-specific T cells bound to cognate DCs. Since stable binding between the T cell and DC required both rules to be satisfied, we then sought to further probe which of these two rules were not being satisfied and preventing the remaining ~15% of antigen-specific T cells from stably binding. To determine whether the velocity rule was causing the incomplete T cell binding, we removed the velocity requirement altogether, and allowed T cells to bind to a DC as long as it met the distance requirement. Under these conditions, the majority (94.5 ± 5.0%) of the antigen-specific T cells stably bound to DCs within the compartment (Table 4.2). Although physiologically motivated, the velocity cut-off is somewhat arbitrary, as we demonstrate experimentally in subsequent sections, T cells moving at much faster velocities are also captured inside the device.

Furthermore, to determine if any improvements could be made by changing the MC packing, while maintaining the same overall DC density, we ran simulations in which the compartment was packed with both large (coated with DCs) and small (uncoated) diameter MCs, thereby decreasing the porosity, and decreasing the average distance between T cells and DCs (Fig 4.4). However, the addition of the small MCs did not materially affect the percentage of stably bound T cells; the remaining 5% of cells (in the absence of a velocity cut-off) likely remain uncaptured due to channelized flow near the boundaries (Table 4.2). This is a limitation of the device and further geometric optimization must be completed in order to minimize this loss.

Table 4.2: Selection of antigen-specific T cells using the computational simple stopping model

	100 big beads	100 big beads + 150 small beads
Velocity cut off: 15 µm/min	84.7 ± 2.5%	86.3 ± 3.8%
No velocity cut off	94.5 ± 5.0%	95.6 ± 4.1%

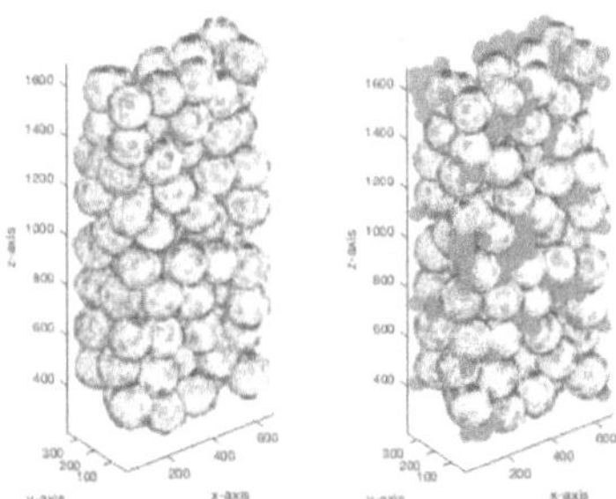

Figure 4.4: Computational simulation of the compartment filled with (left) large MCs (coated with DCs) alone and (right) large MCs (coated with DCs) and small MCs (uncoated).

4.3.3.2 Model 2 – T cell signal integration model

In this section, we removed the velocity cut-off and instead implemented a model based on stimulation. This model has been proposed to explain how antigen-specific T cells transition from transient to stable interactions [40], which inherently accounts for the fact that slower moving T cells have a higher likelihood of binding than quickly moving T cells, without explicitly implementing a velocity-related rule.

In the T cell signal integration model, we assume that as a T cell comes in close contact (<27.5um) with a DC, it will receive some amount of signal from the DC, and that the T cell will bind to the DC above some signal threshold. Fig 4.3d shows an example simulation in which antigen-specific T cells (red) and non-antigen specific T cells (green) are injected at the inlet; most of the non-antigen specific T cells flow to the outlet, while the majority of the antigen-specific T cells become trapped within the device. As a sanity check, we can quantify parameters in the simulations that are commonly used to differentiate between cognate and non-cognate T cell – DCs, such as speed and interaction time. As expected, we find that cognate T cells have a lower speed and make more long-term interactions with DCs than non-cognate T cells (Fig 4.5).

99

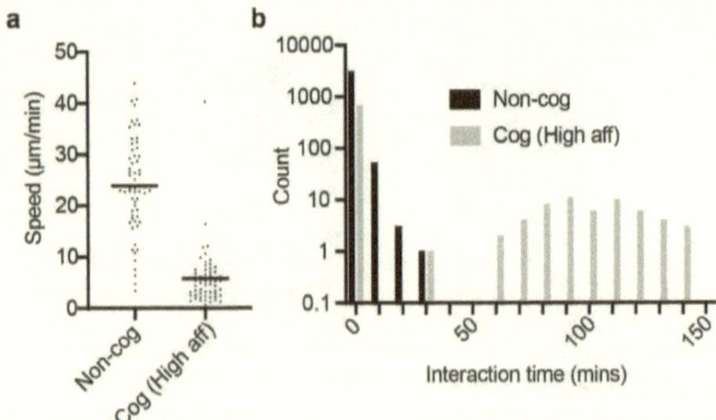

Figure 4.5: Verification of appropriate T cell – DC dynamics in the computational T cell signal integration model. (a-b) The model simulates the expected differences between cognate and non-cognate T cell – DCs in terms of (a) speed and (b) interaction time.

An important use case of this model is to be able to quantify the selection efficiency of antigen-specific T cells. Although the exact parameters used here are not calibrated to our experiments, the following demonstrates the ability to use this type of model to optimize selection efficiency for T cells with varying TCR-pMHC affinities, and even by the varying the flow rate.

First, we assess the selection of antigen-specific T cells as a function of the TCR-pMHC affinity, as we can simulate the selection of high affinity and low affinity antigen-specific T cells by maintaining a constant stimulation threshold, and varying the amount of signal received by the T cell as it contacts a DC, depending on the affinity. Higher affinity T cells receive more signal, thereby reaching the stimulation threshold and transitioning to stable bonds faster than lower affinity T cells. In particular, we find that, while around 96% of both high and low affinity T cells interact with DCs (meaning that they come in close contact with or transiently interact with DCs), 91% of high affinity T cells transition to stable interactions with DCs, and only 72% of low affinity T cells transition to stable interactions (Table 4.3).

We also used the model to determine the percentage of (high affinity) cognate T cells selected by varying the flow rate imposed at the inlet. As the flow rate was increased, although the majority of cognate T cells continue to interact with DCs, the percentage of antigen-specific T cells that stably interact with DCs decreases (Fig 4.6). This is aligned with the notion that *in vivo*, T cells are balancing the need to encounter many different DCs in search of the cognate one, with the need to remain in a location for long enough for the TCR to receive activating signals from pMHC complexes on DCs [144]. By increasing the flow rate, we are ensuring that T cells can encounter numerous DCs, which would be beneficial in terms of screening more T cells, faster; however, they are not remaining in contact with DCs for long enough to receive the appropriate signals. This allows one to tune the screening speed at the cost of selection efficiency. With that being said, we find that by doubling the flow rate, from 0.002 µL/min to 0.004 µL/min, the majority of the antigen-specific T cells still become trapped within the device.

Table 4.3: Selection of antigen-specific T cells using the computational T cell signal integration model, as a function of TCR-pMHC affinity.

TCR affinity	% of cognate T cells that interact with DCs	% of cognate T cells that bind to DCs
High affinity	96 ± 3%	91 ± 5%
Low affinity	96 ± 1%	72 ± 5%

It is important to note that these selection efficiencies are specific to these particular parameters, as well as this particular device (in terms of device dimensions, number of DCs and MCs...) and changing these parameters would change the results. Ideally, one would precisely calibrate the *in silico* model using experimentally measured parameters; nonetheless, with physiologically motivated parameters, we can still estimate how deviations in these parameters, as well as others, such as the degree of bead packing, T cell density, degree of DC confluency and device dimensions can affect the selection efficiency of antigen-specific T cells.

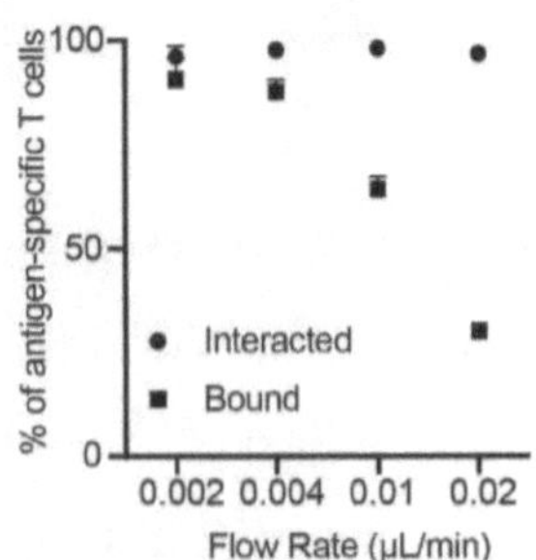

Figure 4.6: Quantification of T cell selection using the T cell signal integration model as a function of T cell flow rate.

We can also use the model to probe similarities between the device and the native lymph node in terms of the numbers of interactions between T cells and DCs. For example, when we simulated injecting WT (non-cognate) T cells in the device at a scaled up cell density of 10×10^6 cells/mL, each T cell interacted with an average of 22 DCs in 2.5 hours, while in mice it has been reported that each non-cognate CD8$^+$ T cell interacts with ~310 DCs during each LN passage, which typically lasts 8-24 hours [132]. We can use the model to make quantitative comparisons which would be difficult to do with experiments alone.

Thus, we can use the CFD-ABM to advise device design to assess T cell selection as a function of different input parameters such as flow rate, geometry and TCR-pMHC affinity, and to make quantitative comparisons at the cellular level.

4.3.4 Microfluidic device

4.3.4.1 Verification of the model system of antigen-specific T cells

Throughout this chapter, we use CD8$^+$ T cells from OT-I TCR transgenic mice interacting either with un-pulsed (non-cognate) or N4 peptide-presenting (cognate) DCs. As shown in chapter 3, OT-I T cells exhibit a slower speed in the presence of cognate N4-presenting DCs in comparison to un-pulsed DCs. Using the same experimental set up as chapter 3, in which the T cells were cultured with cognate or non-cognate DCs under static conditions in a well-plate system, here we assess T cell arrest by quantifying the arrest coefficient, which is the percentage of time a cell has a speed less than 2 µm/min. In Fig 4.7 we show that the arrest coefficient is significantly higher for cognate T cells in comparison to non-cognate T cells. Despite the significant difference in arrest coefficient between cognate and non-cognate T cells, non-cognate T cells still spent 50% of their time in a stationary state under static co-culture conditions.

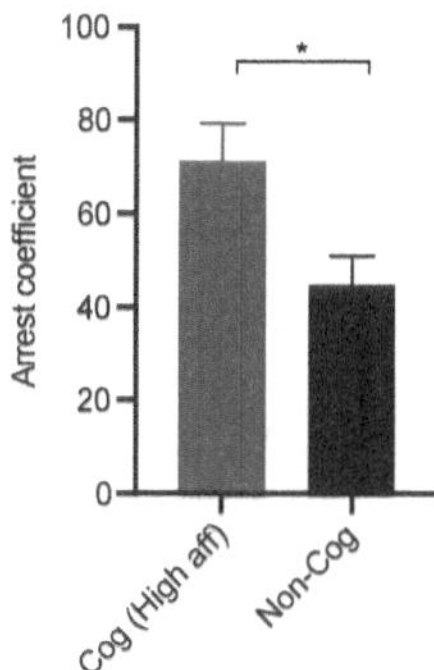

Figure 4.7 Arrest coefficient of cognate or non-cognate T cell – DCs (mean ± standard deviation, t-test)

In order to determine if external forces could help further differentiate stationary cells, we assessed the ability to detach cognate or non-cognate T cells from a 2D monolayer of DCs under successively faster flow. We hypothesized that non-cognate T cells would be detached from DCs at a lower flow rate due to the weaker, and more transient interactions between them in comparison to cognate T cell – DCs. Briefly, we cultured a monolayer of un-pulsed or N4 peptide-presenting DCs in a microfluidic channel, introduced T cells into the channel, and let the T cells interact with DCs under static conditions for 1-2 hours. To assess T cell detachment under flow, we performed time-lapse imaging as we flowed media through the chip at increasingly higher flow rates (Fig 4.8a). One immediately noticeable result is that after 1-2 hours of static culture in channels with cognate T cells and DCs, the majority of T cells had bound to, or were in close contact with, DCs, which was not the case for channels with non-cognate cells. Upon initiating flow, in channels with cognate cells, there were very few T cells which flowed into the imaged region from upstream, whereas in channels with non-cognate cells, many T cells flowed through the imaged region that originated from upstream. We can therefore infer that even in areas upstream of the imaged region, the majority of the cognate T cells had bound to DCs, while the majority of non-cognate T cells had not. We then quantified the percentage of T cells remaining after each successive flow rate was applied (calculated by counting the number of cells remaining, as a percentage of the number of cells at the initial time point). As expected, we found that in the non-cognate and T cell alone devices, around half of the T cells were removed or detached after applying a flow rate of 20 µL/min, whereas for the cog devices, the majority of the T cells stayed attached throughout the whole experiment (Fig 4.8b). This suggests that the cognate T cells make stronger interactions with DCs than the non-cognate cells. However, ~40-50% of the non-cognate T cells did remain within the device even after the highest flow rate, which implies that there will be some degree of non-specific binding within the proposed device. As delineated below, future work involves implementing techniques to reduce non-specific binding (for example by culturing the DCs with anti-CD40 antibodies as in Chapter 3), or integrating a downstream microfluidic device to separate out non-specific T cells from antigen-specific T cells based on the expression of activation markers.

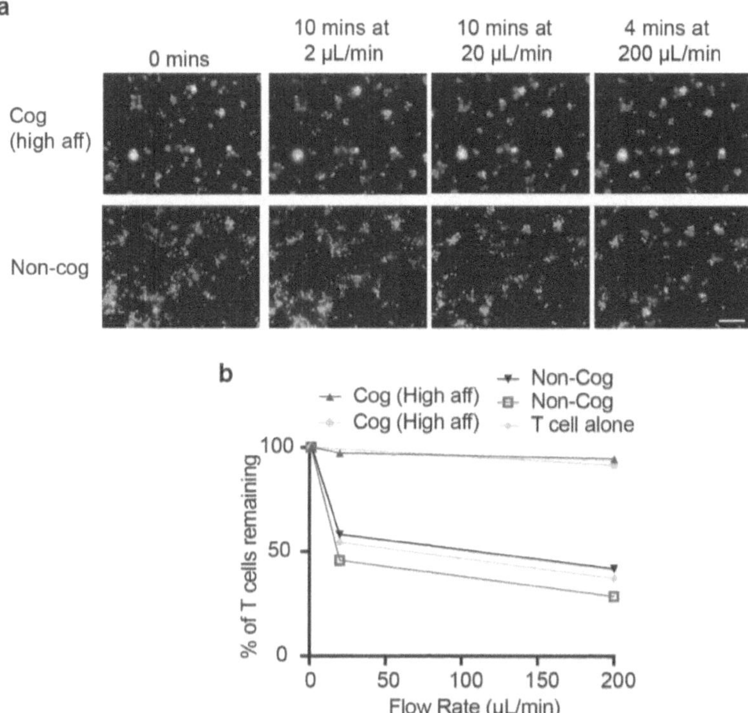

Figure 4.8: T cell detachment in a 2D microfluidic device. (a) T cells (green) were incubated with a 2D monolayer of DCs (red) in a microfluidic device, under static conditions, for 1-2 hours, after which media was flowed through the device at progressively higher flow rates. (Scale bar is 100 µm). (b) The percentage of T cells remaining in the microfluidic device after applying increasing flow rates (normalized to the number of T cells at the initial time point)

4.3.4.2 Microfluidic device fabrication

In order to fabricate microfluidic devices for this application, we went through many iterations of designs, as well as fabrication methods. The first device design iteration was fabricated using acrylic and conventional machining technologies, including laser cutting and CNC milling. This provided the benefit of being able to rapidly prototype the design. In this first iteration, two pieces of acrylic which were engraved with the channel, inlet and outlet, were adhered together, with a cell strainer (75 µm mesh size) sandwiched between two pieces at the outlet. The cell

strainer was sealed with a micro-O ring to trap polystyrene microcarrier beads of diameter 125-

212 µm diameter within the compartment (Fig 4.9). However, we experienced difficulties in

sterilizing these devices using conventional techniques such as autoclaving (acrylic is not

autoclavable) or soaking in ethanol (alcohol dissolved the adhesive material which bonded the

two layers together). Also, gas exchange is required to maintain cell viability for up to 24 hours,

which was not possible using acrylic.

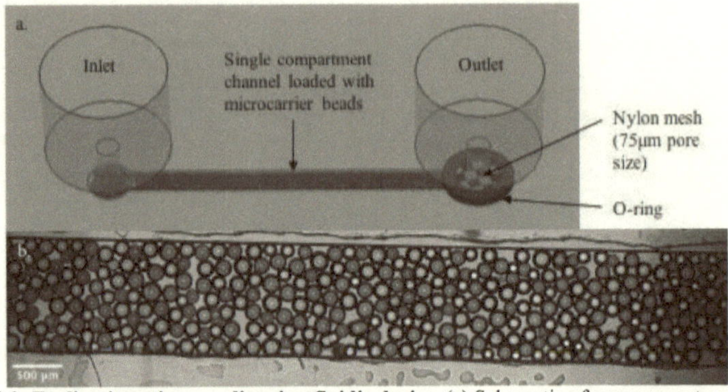

Figure 4.9: Earliest iteration acrylic microfluidic device. (a) Schematic of one-compartment acrylic
device. (b) Trapped polystyrene MCs within the device.

As such, the following iterations of the device were fabricated in PDMS, which is commonly

used for biocompatibility due to the increased gas permeability. Furthermore, valves can be

easily integrated into PDMS microfluidic devices to control fluid flow through the device.

However, conventional methods of fabricating PDMS microfluidic devices using soft

lithography are tedious and not amenable to rapid prototyping. As such, we instead developed

3D-printed molds, which could be readily prototyped, to cast our PDMS devices. However, one

of the issues with 3D printing is the ability to print features of small resolution, as a result, we

experienced difficulties in fabricating devices with features small enough to trap the MCs. This was especially problematic for the soft hydrogel Cytodex 3 MCs which could deform and fit

through the outlet channels, unlike the stiffer polystyrene MCs, the majority of which remained

trapped within the device. In order to 3D print devices with features small enough (<100 μm

channel width) to be able to trap the Cytodex 3 MCs, we tested devices fabricated from molds

printed using a variety of different materials and two different 3D printers: the Stratasys Objet 30

Pro 3D printer and the Asiga Max X 35 stereolithography 3D printer. The Objet 30 Pro was

consistently unable to print 100 μm channels, as the molded PDMS had channels larger than 200

μm in width, allowing the MCs to easily pass through (Fig 4.10a). We then assessed a series of

resins for the Max X 35, including DentaModel Tan, Pro3dure Gr-1 Clear, Pro3dure Gr-10

Black, and the Fun To Do Industrial Blend Black resin. We found optimal resolution using the

Fun To Do Industrial Blend Black resin, as it could reproducibly print molds of channels that

were <100 μm in width. However, we found that under specific circumstances, it was possible

for some MCs to deform and clog the channels (Fig 4.10b). Since we could not 3D print posts at

the outlet due to limitations in the resolution of the 3D printer, we instead designed the device to

have three 100 μm channels at the outlet, to prevent clogging of the whole chip if an MC was

able to pass through one of the three outlet channels (Fig 4.10c).

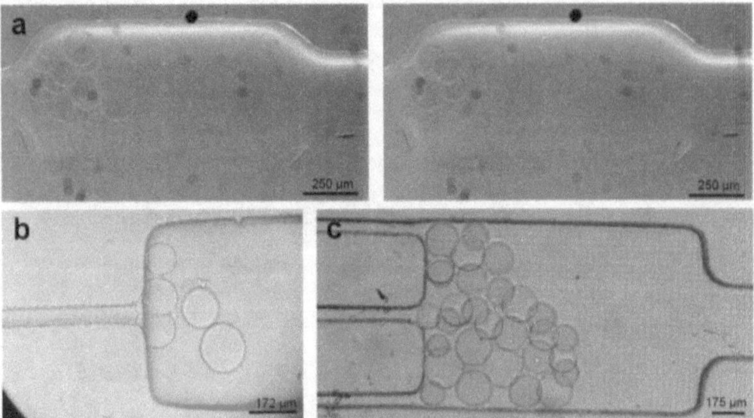

Figure 4.10: PDMS microfluidic devices fabricated using 3D printed molds. (a) PDMS devices were initially fabricated from molds 3D printed on the Stratasys Objet 30 Pro. However, the outlet channel was not as small as intended, and so the Cytodex 3 MCs that collected in the device (left), eventually passed through the outlet (right). (b) PDMS devices with appropriate features were then fabricated from molds 3D printed on the Asiga Max X 35 3D printer, but clogging of the single outlet channel was possible, depending on how the MCs entered the compartment. (c) PDMS devices were then fabricated similarly to (b), but with 3 outlet channels to ensure the device could be used even if one channel was clogged. (In all of the panels, the outlet channel(s) is on the left, and the inlet is on the right)

4.3.4.3 Microcarrier (MC) beads

Next, we assessed DC attachment to two different types of commercially available MCs: polystyrene MCs, and Cytodex 3 MCs (dextran beads coupled to a thin layer of denatured collagen on the surface). After incubating DCs with the (uncoated or fibronectin-coated) MCs overnight, we found that the uncoated Cytodex 3 MCs resulted in the greatest degree of DC attachment (Fig 4.11a). As such, all subsequent experiments were conducted using the uncoated Cytodex 3 MCs. It was not unexpected that the fibronectin-coated Cytodex 3 MCs had reduced DC attachment, because we often found that the MCs aggregated together, which likely prevented DC attachment.

An issue we encountered when flowing and trapping the (Cytodex 3) MCs into the microfluidic device was the inability to consistently fill the compartment with MCs. We eventually realized that when the MCs were suspended in PBS, they rapidly settled within the syringe, which then clogged the needle, precluding their injection into the device. The rate at which the MCs settle, the settling velocity, is a function of particle density, fluid density, particle radius and the dynamic viscosity. Therefore, one way to reduce the settling velocity is to increase the viscosity of the fluid that the MCs were suspended in [151]. As such, we compared the efficiency of injecting Cytodex 3 MCs suspended in fluids of varying viscosity - PBS, PBS supplemented with 0.5% low viscosity methyl cellulose, or PBS supplemented with 0.5% high viscosity methyl cellulose. Consistent with our hypothesis, we found that increasing the viscosity of the suspending solution resulted in increased filling of the channel (Fig 4.11b-d). Importantly, we found that changing the fluid viscosity did not affect DC attachment to the MCs, despite the increased shear stress associated with the increased viscosity (Fig 4.11e). Although some MCs were more confluent than others, the distribution of confluency was also apparent prior to injection (Fig 4.11a) and likely not caused by injecting the MCs into the microfluidic device.

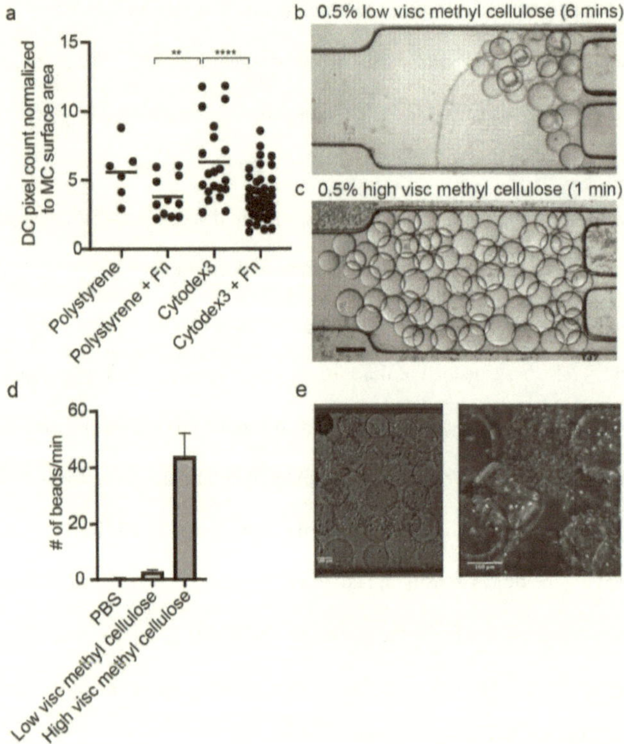

Figure 4.11: Optimization of MC conditions. (a) Quantification of DC attachment to different types of MCs (n>6, mean, One-way ANOVA with Bonferroni's *post-hoc*). (b-c) Images of uncoated Cytodex 3 MCs suspended in (b) 0.5% low viscosity methyl cellulose and injected into the device at 30 μL/min for 6 minutes or (c) 0.5% high viscosity methyl cellulose and injected into the device at 30 μL/min for 1 minute (scale bar is 200 μm). (d) Quantification of (b-c, n=2, mean ± standard deviation). (e) Confocal images of Cytodex 3 MCs coated with DCs (purple) which were suspended in 0.5% high viscosity methyl cellulose and injected into a microfluidic device (scale bar is 100 μm).

4.3.4.4 Integration of components

After testing and optimizing each individual component, including the model system of antigen-specific T cells and corresponding DCs, the microfluidic device, and the microcarrier beads, the final step was to combine the various components and assess the ability to use the integrated device to select antigen-specific T cells. We first assessed the selection of OT-I CD8+ T cells in a device packed with Cytodex 3 MCs coated with N4-DCs, and observed that the T cells (green) stably arrested on cognate DCs (black arrows in Fig 4.12a). Importantly, upon closer examination, the majority of the T cells that were stationary within the device were interacting with DCs, and not simply binding to the MCs. In Fig 4.12b, we show an example of a T cell which momentarily stops on an empty area of the MC, but rapidly detaches.

We then compared the selection of OT-I (cognate) CD8$^+$ T cells and WT B6 (non-cognate) CD8$^+$ T cells simultaneously, in a device packed with MCs coated with N4-DCs. By assessing the selection of cognate and non-cognate T cells in the same device, the results from that device are internally normalized to the number of DCs, which could influence the number of stably bound T cells. We injected the T cells through the device at a flow rate of 0.5 µL/min, which corresponds to an interstitial velocity of ~6 mm/min, which is orders of magnitude higher than the intended speed, and higher than what was initially tested in the ABM. In Fig 4.12c, we show the accumulation of cognate and non-cognate T cells within 3 different microfluidic devices, in a single plane. In all three devices, we see a more rapid accumulation of cognate T cells in comparison to the non-cognate T cells. However, we observed some subtle differences between the experiments, including the overall amount of cells bound, and the rate at which cells have accumulated. These variabilities could be attributed to differences in the number of DCs per device (due to differences in DC confluency on the MCs), the plane imaged, or differences in the number of T cells that were injected (potentially due to settling within the syringe over time). Curiously, in two of the experiments (Fig 4.12c (middle and right)), we observed a decrease in the number of accumulating T cells. However, this is likely due to photobleaching, or T cells moving out of the plane over time, which can lead to undercounting at late times. Nonetheless, we have demonstrated the ability to use this type of device, which leverages the interaction

dynamics between T cells and cognate vs non-cognate DCs, to preferentially select for antigen-

specific T cells.

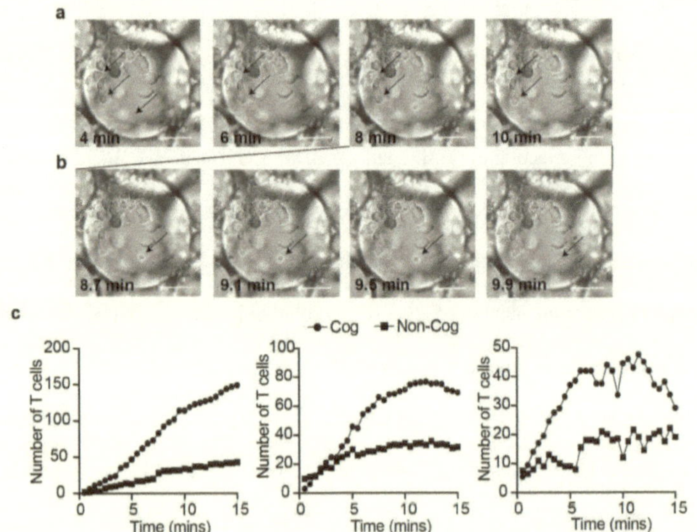

Figure 4.12: Accumulation of cognate T cells within the one-compartment device.
(a-b) Time-lapse images of cognate T cells flowing through a microfluidic device packed with DC-N4-
coated MCs. The arrows in (a) denote T cells attaching to DCs, and the arrows in (b) denote a T cell
which briefly binds to empty space on the MC but quickly detaches (scale bar is 50 μm) (c)
Quantification of cognate (OT-I) T cell or non-cognate (B6) T cell accumulation (in one plane), in three
devices packed with DC-N4-coated MCs.

4.3.4.5 Valves

Although we did not incorporate valves into the current unidirectional, one-compartment device,

future iterations with multiple compartments and both horizontal and vertical flow will require

the integration of valves. In anticipation of this, we modified previously developed screw valves

for future integration [1, 152]. These torque-actuated valves control fluid flow by compressing a

thin PDMS membrane which collapses the channel. Screw valves have many advantages to the widely used pneumatic valves [153], including their ease of fabrication, use, and integration into microfluidic devices, as well as their ability to close channels with rectangular, circular and semi-circular cross-sectional areas [152].

Specifically, we modified the pre-fabricated screw valves developed by Hulme et al. [1], which have three PDMS layers, with the screw held in place with an epoxy. Incorporation of the valves into the channel involves first coating the channel mold with a thin layer of PDMS, and then manually positioning the valve over the channel-of-interest. The channel and valves are then cast with PDMS to crosslink the valves in place, and form the microfluidic device. In order to simplify the design and secure the screw to ensure its ability to consistently compress the PDMS membrane and flow channel, we fabricated a 2-layer PDMS valve, comprised of a PDMS membrane bound to a second PDMS layer with a nut enclosed within it (Fig 4.13a). In our modified design, the screw could be inserted into and securely held in place by the PDMS and nut to maintain its vertical orientation and ensure turning the screw compressed the membrane uniformly. Another limitation we encountered with the pre-fabricated screw valves was difficulties in aligning them with the appropriate channel, because if the valve moved slightly during crosslinking of the PDMS, then the valve would not properly function. To overcome this, we first attempted to incorporate grooves in the mold to facilitate screw valve alignment (Fig 4.13b). Although the valves were often functional in this configuration (for example, they were able to isolate the two compartments as seen in Fig 4.14b), the grooves did not consistently prevent shifting during crosslinking. In order to minimize shift in each of the individual valves, we fabricated a single piece containing all of the valves, and then to ensure proper alignment over the channels, we incorporated alignment holes and pillars into the PDMS piece and the 3D printed mold, respectively (Fig 4.13c). This ensured that all of the valves maintained their position during crosslinking and were able to consistently control fluid flow through the appropriate channel. These combined pre-fabricated valves could be integrated into future iterations of the multi-compartment device.

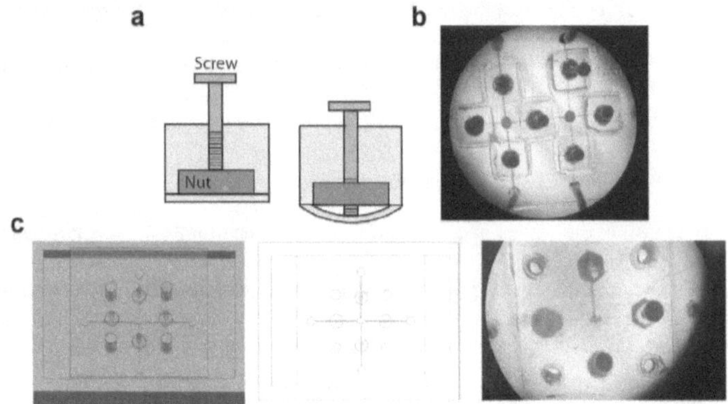

Figure 4.13: Screw valves. (a) Schematic diagram of the pre-fabricated screw valves modified from [1] (b) Individual screw valves positioned over the channels in a 2-compartment device using alignment grooves (c) 4 screw valves were fabricated in one piece, and positioned over the channels in a 1-compartment device using alignment holes and posts (SolidWorks schematics in left and middle, fabricated device in right) (The screw has a diameter of 1mm).

4.4 Discussion

In this chapter, we developed an artificial microfluidic lymph node to select antigen-specific T cells, in order to overcome two main issues with current T cell selection devices: the ability to screen a large number of T cells, and the ability to test a mixed population of T cells against a library of antigens. To overcome these limitations, we aimed to mimic some of the features of the T cell zone of the lymph node that enable the efficient selection of antigen-specific cells *in vivo*. First, we recapitulate the architecture of the T cell zone of the LN by creating a sessile network of antigen-presenting DCs, which are scanned by migrating T cells. As the T cells interact with DCs, cognate interactions will result in stable, long-term interactions, whereas non-cognate interactions will result in transient interactions. Ultimately, this leads to the trapping of predominantly antigen-specific T cells within the device. Using agent-based simulations and experiments, we demonstrate that this structural organization facilitates T cell interactions with DCs, and we observe a preferential accumulation of cognate, antigen-specific T cells, in comparison to non-antigen-specific T cells in a one-compartment device. Furthermore, we could scale up both device dimensions, and T cell density to screen millions of T cells within 24 hours, as demonstrated analytically. Finally, *in vivo*, each T cell interacts with many DCs presenting many different antigens, thus, the rationale behind this compartment-based device was to be able to screen a mixed population of T cells against a library of antigens, to increase the probability of encountering the cognate pMHC. Although we did not demonstrate this experimentally, the current one-compartment device could be scaled-up to screen against multiple antigens.

Although further work is required to fully develop this biomimetic microfluidic device, here, we demonstrate the ability to leverage the stable binding interactions between T cells and DCs to preferentially select and trap flowing antigen-specific T cells on cognate DCs. Once scaled up, we identify two main impacts that this device will have on cell therapies: 1. Improving the therapeutic efficacy of TCR-engineered T cell therapies, by increasing the probability of identifying potentially clinically relevant T cells and 2. Simplifying the selection process to facilitate the scale-up and scale-out of cell manufacturing process. Microfluidic devices can be automated, precisely controlled, and integrated with upstream or downstream processes, thereby simplifying and streamlining a critical step in the manufacturing of certain adoptive T cell therapies.

Chapter 5: Conclusion and Future Directions

5.1 Conclusion

As more cell therapies become approved and commercialized, moving from the bench to the clinic, an emerging issue is how to manufacture these extremely personalized, often one batch products in a cost-effective, reproducible manner, despite complex processes, as well as patient-to-patient variability in both the raw materials, and the yield. For example, in order to reduce costs associated with centralized manufacturing of CAR-T cell therapies (which cost ~$475,000 [154]), technologies such as Miltenyi's CliniMACS Prodigy have been developed to separate, activate, transduce and expand T cells in an integrated, all-in-one device, to potentially manufacture CAR-T cells at the point-of-care or in a decentralized facility, in a standardized manner. In order for cell therapies, especially personalized autologous therapies, to be available to all of the patients who would benefit from them, further improvements must be made in their manufacturing processes, in terms of reproducibility, scalability, simplicity and cost-effectiveness. This book demonstrates the use of three different technologies to improve cell therapy manufacturing:

1. Alginate microwell hydrogel scaffolds to fabricate therapeutic pre-vascularized organoids in a reproducible, controllable and scalable manner.
2. Deep learning-based approach to rapidly classify antigen-specific T cells.
3. Biomimetic microfluidic artificial lymph node to select antigen-specific T cells.

In Chapter 1, we leverage the non-adhesive, and dynamic crosslinking properties of alginate to create microwell scaffolds to help improve the reproducibility and scalability of 3D organoid-based cell therapies. In particular, we demonstrate the ability to control the size and structure of pre-vascularized organoids comprised of ECs and MSCs as a function of the cell source, ratio of cells, or size of the microwells. Furthermore, by uncrosslinking the alginate scaffold, the organoids can be harvested in a gentle manner without damaging their structure or impairing their functionality. Although the pre-vascularized organoids produced using the alginate microwells did not significantly improve therapeutic outcomes in comparison to single cell suspensions in a mouse model of hindlimb ischemia, we did observe an improvement in comparison to saline alone. Nonetheless, the alginate microwell scaffolds are a platform technology that can be used to improve the manufacturability of many different types of organoid-based cell therapies.

In Chapters 2 and 3 we switch our focus to T cell therapies, which require cost-effective and scalable methods to facilitate their clinical translation. In particular, the selection of antigen-specific T cells is a critical step in the development of TCR-engineered T cells, as the TCR on the identified antigen-specific T cells can be sequenced, and specific populations of host T cells can be engineered to express the TCR-of-interest. This would be especially relevant if the antigen-specific T cells are identified from donor T cells. However, most assays used to select antigen-specific T cells, including those used in clinical trials, are inefficient, and would be difficult to adapt for large-scale manufacturing, and widespread use. Furthermore, although TCR-engineered T cell therapies have great potential, their therapeutic efficacy is still limited; one potential reason for this limited efficacy is the inability of conventional assays to select T cells with anti-tumor reactivity against all potentially clinically relevant tumor antigens. As such, here, we develop two methods which overcome these limitations. In Chapter 2, we develop a deep learning model which can rapidly classify different types of high and low affinity CD8$^+$ T cells. In Chapter 3, we develop a microfluidic "lymph node", which was inspired by the T cell

zone of the lymph node with the aim of screening a mixed population of T cells against libraries

of antigens to improve the sensitivity and accuracy of T cell selection. Ultimately, the purpose of

both of these technologies (deep learning and microfluidics) was to move towards fully

automated, high-throughput manufacturing processes, to reduce the need for complex and time-,

resource- and labor- intensive processes, and to improve the therapeutic efficacy.

5.2 Future directions

Future work is required in order to further demonstrate the applications, and achieve the full

potential of each of the three technologies discussed in this book.

5.2.1 Therapeutic efficacy of pre-vascularized organoids fabricated using the alginate scaffold

Though we demonstrate improvements in the manufacturing of organoids, more work is needed

to demonstrate the functional improvements achieved with pre-vascularized organoids in

comparison to single cells. To do so, future work involves optimizing the surgery model, and the

in vitro organoid culture conditions. In particular, in the next study, recovery will be assessed in

a more severe ischemic injury model in which the femoral artery will be ligated and excised from

the distal site of the deep femoral bifurcation to a site just distal to the popliteal/saphenous

bifurcation, known as the A-strip model [78]. Goto et al. demonstrated that the A-strip injury

consistently resulted in toe necrosis within 14 days, indicating that it is more severe than our

initial injury model, in which no necrosis was observed. By inducing a more severe ischemic

injury, it is possible that cell replacement would be the dominant form of recovery, in which case the pre-vascularized nature of the organoids is hypothesized to be more beneficial in inducing recovery than single cells. Alternatively, rather than inducing ischemia in C57BL/6 mice, we could instead use BALB/c mice, which have been reported to experience a more profound ischemic response, and recover more slowly, likely due to variations in pre-existing collateral arteries [155]. Other parameters that will require optimizing to improve therapeutic efficacy include organoid dosage, as well as *in vitro* culture conditions. For example, culturing the organoids longer *in vitro*, could enable further organization and maturation prior to *in vivo* delivery; however, the resulting organoid diameter would have to be closely monitored to ensure that it less than 150 μm, to stay within the diffusion limit of oxygen and nutrients.

5.2.2 Other uses of the alginate microwell scaffold platform technology

The alginate microwell scaffolds are a platform technology that can be used to fabricate many types of cellular aggregates, for instance, vascularized beta cells to treat Type 1 diabetes. Current islet transplantation methods are impeded by cellular degradation soon after transplantation [156], and so improvements are needed to extend the therapeutic effects of insulin-secreting cells and create a lasting cellular network.

5.2.3 Improvements to the deep learning-based approach to classify cognate and non-cognate T cell – DCs

A number of improvements can be made to both the video processing workflow, and the deep learning model to improve the classifier's ability to predict whether a T cell is making cognate or non-cognate interactions with a DC.

5.2.3.1 Improvements to the video processing workflow

Since this model classifies videos of T cells as they interact with DCs, it is essential that the T cell tracks are generated accurately, and that each video is indeed following the same T cell. Although the automated cell tracking software is accurate for the most part, there were few cases where the T cells were not tracked properly, and it was clear that the same T cell was not being followed the entire time. As such, we had to manually discard those inaccurately tracked T cells to ensure the reliability of the videos. Future work could involve using more accurate methods, for example deep learning [157], to track the T cells.

Another limitation associated with video processing is accurate thresholding of the cells. In our approach, it is necessary for both the T cells and DCs to be correctly thresholded, to make an accurate classification. Due to the strong staining of the T cells (using calcein), they were consistently thresholded accurately. However, due to the diffuse staining within the dendrites of the DCs (using a cell tracker), the DC thresholding was more inconsistent. Thus, future work involves improving the DC staining process to ensure that the whole DC can be accurately binarized.

Furthermore, since we are currently generating videos in the frame of reference of the T cells, we lose spatial information such as how far the T cells are moving, or the velocity with which they are moving. Future work involves generating the videos in alternative ways, such as by reducing the magnification, and following the T cell in the lab frame of reference, rather than the frame of reference of the T cells.

5.2.3.2 Improvements to the deep learning model

Currently, we demonstrate the generalizability of the model by training it using videos of OT-I T cells, and then testing it on videos of the same cells, NY8.3 T cells, and OT-I T cells making low affinity interactions. In order to improve the generalizability of the model, future work involves training a model with a variety of CD8$^+$ T cell types. Increasing the size of the training data set and including different types of CD8$^+$ T cells would likely further improve the generalizability and fidelity of the model.

We also show that the model trained on the CD8$^+$ T cells did not generalize well to the CD4$^+$ T cells. Although in the past most cell therapies have involved the delivery of CD8$^+$ T cells, due to their ability to directly kill target cells when differentiated into their cytotoxic effector forms, it has become increasingly clear that CD4$^+$ T cells are also necessary to effectively treat cancer. Also, regulatory T cells therapies, such as for Type 1 diabetes or other autoimmune diseases, would require the selection CD4$^+$ T cells. As such, future work involves training a separate binary classifier using videos of CD4$^+$ T cells in order to classify cognate and non-cognate CD4$^+$ T cells.

Furthermore, here, we use anti-CD40 antibodies to amplify the differences between cognate and non-cognate T cells, by increasing contact between cognate T cells and DCs, and decreasing non-specific binding by non-cognate T cells and DCs. Future work involves implementing other mechanisms to further differentiate between cognate and non-cognate T cell – DC interactions, for example by introducing low levels of flow into the system, or by introducing other potentially blocking antibodies.

5.2.4 Integration of the deep learning model with a microfluidic cell sorting device

Finally, thus far, we demonstrate the ability of the deep learning model to classify videos of T cells. However, in order to select the T cells classified as being cognate, future work involves integrating the model into a microfluidic cell sorting device. An example of a microfluidic cell sorting device which is modeled after Segaliny et al. [103] would be to confine CD8$^+$ T cell – DC pairs within microdroplets, which can be docked. Following continuous monitoring of the microdroplets, those that are classified as having cognate T cells by the deep learning model could be selectively released, and the T cells could be isolated for downstream processes, such as functional assays.

5.2.5 Further development of the microfluidic artificial lymph node

In order to further understand the capabilities of this device to select antigen-specific T cells, additional experiments can be performed. For instance, T cell selection should be assessed as a function of flow rate. Although we initially sought to flow the T cells through the device at an interstitial velocity of 15 µm/min (corresponding to the average velocity in the lymph node, and as was implemented in the CFD-ABM), experimentally, we find that antigen-specific T cells can make stable interactions with cognate DCs at much higher velocities. As such, further work is required to determine the optimal flow rate and T cell velocity to maximize the selection efficiency and throughput, while minimizing non-specific binding. Furthermore, in order to understand the sensitivity and specificity of the device, antigen-specific T cells should be spiked into non-antigen-specific T cells at different concentrations. Although we demonstrate selection of antigen-specific T cells in a 1:1 mixed population (antigen-specific to WT B6 T cells), in order to assess the ability to select very rare antigen-specific T cells, a much more skewed population must be tested. Importantly, to test the ability of this proposed device to screen a mixed population T cells against multiple antigens, the number of compartments and parallel channels should be scaled up. In doing so, the addition of many compartments may also require a more complex flow control system, such as Quake valves. Furthermore, this device should eventually be tested using both $CD4^+$ and $CD8^+$ T cells, as well as patient samples, and the selection efficiency should be compared to the conventional assays and devices described in Table 4.1.

5.2.6 Calibrating the ABM

In order to improve the utility of the ABM, the specific interaction parameters should be calibrated using experimental observations. For example, by determining where the T cells get trapped inside the device, the TCR-pMHC binding signal can be inferred, and input into the model to improve its accuracy. Furthermore, in order to develop a more realistic model, and to accurately recapitulate the experimental results, a number of improvements can be made, such as making the signal intensity a function of both TCR affinity and pMHC density, incorporating signal decay, as well as transient and non-specific interactions. Ultimately, with a more accurate model, more *in silico* optimization of the device can be done.

5.2.7 Reduction of non-specific binding in the microfluidic artificial lymph node

Due to the non-specific binding of non-cognate T cells to DCs, an issue that may limit the utility of the device, despite a potentially high sensitivity, could be a low specificity. Future efforts should focus on reducing non-specific binding without impacting specific binding, potentially by increasing the flow rate (although it is very high as it is). Alternatively, as demonstrated in Chapter 3, the addition of anti-CD40 antibodies reduces long-term interactions between non-cognate T cells and DCs, which could similarly be implemented here.

If significant non-specific binding persists, a downstream device can be integrated to verify the activation of the selected T cells. This is because only the antigen-specific T cells should become activated and display relevant markers, such as CD69, CD154 and/or CD137. The activated T cells could therefore be sorted using magnetic-activated cell sorting [158], fluorescence activated cell sorting [159], or a single cell trapping device from which individual cells can be recovered [160].

References

[1]   S. E. Hulme, S. S. Shevkoplyas, and G. M. Whitesides, "Incorporation of prefabricated screw, pneumatic, and solenoid valves into microfluidic devices," *Lab on a Chip,* vol. 9, no. 1, pp. 79-86, 2009.

[2]   L. L. W. Wang *et al.,* "Cell therapies in the clinic," *Bioengineering & translational medicine,* vol. 6, no. 2, p. e10214, 2021.

[3]   K. Wang *et al.,* "A multiscale simulation framework for the manufacturing facility and supply chain of autologous cell therapies," *Cytotherapy,* vol. 21, no. 10, pp. 1081-1093, 2019.

[4]   N. C. M. Consortium, "Achieving Large-Scale, Cost-Effective, Reproducible Manufacturing of High-Quality Cells: A Technology Roadmap to 2025, 2016," ed.

[5]   P. S. Thakuri, C. Liu, G. D. Luker, and H. Tavana, "Biomaterials-Based Approaches to Tumor Spheroid and Organoid Modeling," *Advanced healthcare materials,* vol. 7, no. 6, p. 1700980, 2018.

[6]   M. Hofer and M. P. Lutolf, "Engineering organoids," *Nature Reviews Materials,* vol. 6, no. 5, pp. 402-420, 2021.

[7]   A. Alajati *et al.,* "Spheroid-based engineering of a human vasculature in mice," *Nat. Methods,* vol. 5, no. 5, pp. 439-45, May 2008, doi: 10.1038/nmeth.1198.

[8]   K. H. Nam, A. S. Smith, S. Lone, S. Kwon, and D. H. Kim, "Biomimetic 3D Tissue Models for Advanced High-Throughput Drug Screening," *J. Lab. Autom.,* vol. 20, no. 3, pp. 201-15, Jun 2015, doi: 10.1177/2211068214557813.

[9]   C. S. Ong *et al.,* "In vivo therapeutic applications of cell spheroids," *Biotechnology advances,* vol. 36, no. 2, pp. 494-505, 2018.

[10]   T. Takebe *et al.,* "Vascularized and functional human liver from an iPSC-derived organ bud transplant," *Nature,* vol. 499, no. 7459, pp. 481-4, Jul 25 2013, doi: 10.1038/nature12271.

[11]   R. Walser, W. Metzger, A. Gorg, T. Pohlemann, M. D. Menger, and M. W. Laschke, "Generation of co-culture spheroids as vascularisation units for bone tissue engineering," *Eur Cell Mater,* vol. 26, pp. 222-33, 2013. [Online]. Available: http://www.ncbi.nlm.nih.gov/pubmed/24197544.

[12]   K. K. Yap *et al.,* "Enhanced liver progenitor cell survival and differentiation in vivo by spheroid implantation in a vascularized tissue engineering chamber," *Biomaterials,* vol. 34, no. 16, pp. 3992-4001, May 2013, doi: 10.1016/j.biomaterials.2013.02.011.

[13]   W. L. Dissanayaka, L. Zhu, K. M. Hargreaves, L. Jin, and C. Zhang, "Scaffold-free Prevascularized Microtissue Spheroids for Pulp Regeneration," *J Dent Res,* vol. 93, no. 12, pp. 1296-303, Dec 2014, doi: 10.1177/0022034514550040.

[14]   F. Verseijden *et al.,* "Prevascular structures promote vascularization in engineered human adipose tissue constructs upon implantation," *Cell Transplant,* vol. 19, no. 8, pp. 1007-20, 2010, doi: 10.3727/096368910X492571.

[15]   U. Meyer, H. P. Wiesmann, J. Libera, R. Depprich, C. Naujoks, and J. Handschel, "Cartilage defect regeneration by ex vivo engineered autologous microtissue--preliminary results," *In Vivo,* vol. 26, no. 2, pp. 251-7, Mar-Apr 2012. [Online]. Available: http://www.ncbi.nlm.nih.gov/pubmed/22351666.

[16]   J. H. Kim, I. S. Park, Y. Park, Y. Jung, S. H. Kim, and S.-H. Kim, "Therapeutic angiogenesis of three-dimensionally cultured adipose-derived stem cells in rat infarcted hearts," *Cytotherapy*, vol. 15, no. 5, pp. 542-556, 2013.

[17]   A. A. Dayem, S. B. Lee, K. Kim, K. M. Lim, T.-i. Jeon, and S.-G. Cho, "Recent advances in organoid culture for insulin production and diabetes therapy: methods and challenges," *BMB reports*, vol. 52, no. 5, p. 295, 2019.

[18]   E. Henry *et al.*, "Adult lung spheroid cells contain progenitor cells and mediate regeneration in rodents with bleomycin-induced pulmonary fibrosis," *Stem cells translational medicine*, vol. 4, no. 11, pp. 1265-1274, 2015.

[19]   C. Eschen *et al.*, "Clinical outcome is significantly better with spheroid-based autologous chondrocyte implantation manufactured with more stringent cell culture criteria," *Osteoarthritis and Cartilage Open*, vol. 2, no. 1, p. 100033, 2020.

[20]   M. Huch, J. A. Knoblich, M. P. Lutolf, and A. Martinez-Arias, "The hope and the hype of organoid research," *Development*, vol. 144, no. 6, pp. 938-941, 2017.

[21]   R. M. Sutherland, J. A. McCredie, and W. R. Inch, "Growth of multicell spheroids in tissue culture as a model of nodular carcinomas," *J Natl Cancer Inst*, vol. 46, no. 1, pp. 113-20, Jan 1971. [Online]. Available: http://www.ncbi.nlm.nih.gov/pubmed/5101993.

[22]   Y. C. Tung, A. Y. Hsiao, S. G. Allen, Y. S. Torisawa, M. Ho, and S. Takayama, "High-throughput 3D spheroid culture and drug testing using a 384 hanging drop array," *Analyst*, vol. 136, no. 3, pp. 473-8, Feb 7 2011, doi: 10.1039/c0an00609b.

[23]   O. Frey, P. M. Misun, D. A. Fluri, J. G. Hengstler, and A. Hierlemann, "Reconfigurable microfluidic hanging drop network for multi-tissue interaction and analysis," *Nat. Commun.*, vol. 5, p. 4250, 2014, doi: 10.1038/ncomms5250.

[24]   S. M. Ehsan, K. M. Welch-Reardon, M. L. Waterman, C. C. Hughes, and S. C. George, "A three-dimensional in vitro model of tumor cell intravasation," *Integr Biol (Camb)*, vol. 6, no. 6, pp. 603-10, Jun 2014, doi: 10.1039/c3ib40170g.

[25]   J. M. Yuhas, A. P. Li, A. O. Martinez, and A. J. Ladman, "A simplified method for production and growth of multicellular tumor spheroids," *Cancer Res*, vol. 37, no. 10, pp. 3639-43, Oct 1977. [Online]. Available: http://www.ncbi.nlm.nih.gov/pubmed/908012.

[26]   W. Metzger *et al.*, "The liquid overlay technique is the key to formation of co-culture spheroids consisting of primary osteoblasts, fibroblasts and endothelial cells," *Cytotherapy*, vol. 13, no. 8, pp. 1000-12, Sep 2011, doi: 10.3109/14653249.2011.583233.

[27]   A. Wenger *et al.*, "Development and characterization of a spheroidal coculture model of endothelial cells and fibroblasts for improving angiogenesis in tissue engineering," *Cells Tissues Organs*, vol. 181, no. 2, pp. 80-8, 2005, doi: 10.1159/000091097.

[28]   H. J. Chung and T. G. Park, "Injectable cellular aggregates prepared from biodegradable porous microspheres for adipose tissue engineering," *Tissue Eng. Part A*, vol. 15, no. 6, pp. 1391-400, Jun 2009, doi: 10.1089/ten.tea.2008.0344.

[29]   D. R. Griffin, W. M. Weaver, P. O. Scumpia, D. Di Carlo, and T. Segura, "Accelerated wound healing by injectable microporous gel scaffolds assembled from annealed building blocks," *Nat. Mater.*, vol. 14, no. 7, pp. 737-44, Jul 2015, doi: 10.1038/nmat4294.

[30]   N. Huebsch *et al.*, "Matrix elasticity of void-forming hydrogels controls transplanted-stem-cell-mediated bone formation," *Nat. Mater.*, vol. 14, no. 12, pp. 1269-77, Dec 2015, doi: 10.1038/nmat4407.

[31]   Y. Li *et al.*, "Primed 3D injectable microniches enabling low-dosage cell therapy for critical limb ischemia," *PNAS*, vol. 111, no. 37, pp. 13511-13516, 2014.

[32]   A. Ovsianikov, A. Khademhosseini, and V. Mironov, "The synergy of scaffold-based and scaffold-free tissue engineering strategies," *Trends Biotechnol.*, vol. 36, no. 4, pp. 348-357, 2018.

[33]   D. R. Fooksman *et al.*, "Functional anatomy of T cell activation and synapse formation," *Annual review of immunology*, vol. 28, pp. 79-105, 2009.

[34]   M. W. Toepke and D. J. Beebe, "PDMS absorption of small molecules and consequences in microfluidic applications," *Lab Chip*, vol. 6, no. 12, pp. 1484-6, Dec 2006, doi: 10.1039/b612140c.

[35]   K. Shimizu *et al.*, "Poly (N-isopropylacrylamide)-coated microwell arrays for construction and recovery of multicellular spheroids," *J Biosci Bioeng*, vol. 115, no. 6, pp. 695-699, 2013.

[36]   H. Tekin, M. Anaya, M. D. Brigham, C. Nauman, R. Langer, and A. Khademhosseini, "Stimuli-responsive microwells for formation and retrieval of cell aggregates," *Lab Chip*, vol. 10, no. 18, pp. 2411-2418, 2010.

[37]   T. Anada *et al.*, "Three-dimensional cell culture device utilizing thin membrane deformation by decompression," *Sensor Actuat B-Chem*, vol. 147, no. 1, pp. 376-379, 2010.

[38]   P. Guermonprez, J. Valladeau, L. Zitvogel, C. Théry, and S. Amigorena, "Antigen presentation and T cell stimulation by dendritic cells," *Annual review of immunology*, vol. 20, no. 1, pp. 621-667, 2002.

[39]   A. Lanzavecchia and F. Sallusto, "Regulation of T cell immunity by dendritic cells," *Cell*, vol. 106, no. 3, pp. 263-266, 2001.

[40]   P. Bousso, "T-cell activation by dendritic cells in the lymph node: lessons from the movies," *Nature Reviews Immunology*, vol. 8, no. 9, pp. 675-684, 2008.

[41]   G. A. Rabinovich, D. Gabrilovich, and E. M. Sotomayor, "Immunosuppressive strategies that are mediated by tumor cells," *Annu. Rev. Immunol.*, vol. 25, pp. 267-296, 2007.

[42]   G. W. Tormoen, M. R. Crittenden, and M. J. Gough, "Role of the immunosuppressive microenvironment in immunotherapy," *Advances in radiation oncology*, vol. 3, no. 4, pp. 520-526, 2018.

[43]   A. E. Zamora, J. C. Crawford, and P. G. Thomas, "Hitting the target: how T cells detect and eliminate tumors," *The Journal of Immunology*, vol. 200, no. 2, pp. 392-399, 2018.

[44]   N. P. Restifo, M. E. Dudley, and S. A. Rosenberg, "Adoptive immunotherapy for cancer: harnessing the T cell response," *Nature Reviews Immunology*, vol. 12, no. 4, pp. 269-281, 2012.

[45]   S. A. Rosenberg *et al.*, "Durable complete responses in heavily pretreated patients with metastatic melanoma using T-cell transfer immunotherapy," *Clinical cancer research*, vol. 17, no. 13, pp. 4550-4557, 2011.

[46]   S. Stevanović *et al.*, "A phase II study of tumor-infiltrating lymphocyte therapy for human papillomavirus–associated epithelial cancers," *Clinical Cancer Research*, vol. 25, no. 5, pp. 1486-1493, 2019.

[47]   R. C. Larson and M. V. Maus, "Recent advances and discoveries in the mechanisms and functions of CAR T cells," *Nature Reviews Cancer*, vol. 21, no. 3, pp. 145-161, 2021.

[48]   A. Mullard, "FDA approves fourth CAR-T cell therapy," *Nature reviews. Drug Discovery*, 2021.

[49]   S. S. Chandran and C. A. Klebanoff, "T cell receptor-based cancer immunotherapy: emerging efficacy and pathways of resistance," *Immunological reviews,* vol. 290, no. 1, pp. 127-147, 2019.

[50]   E. DeW, "Driving T-cell immunotherapy to solid tumors," *Nature biotechnology,* vol. 36, no. 3, p. 215, 2018.

[51]   L. Gaissmaier, M. Elshiaty, and P. Christopoulos, "Breaking bottlenecks for the TCR therapy of cancer," *Cells,* vol. 9, no. 9, p. 2095, 2020.

[52]   V. Leko and S. A. Rosenberg, "Identifying and targeting human tumor antigens for T cell-based immunotherapy of solid tumors," *Cancer Cell,* 2020.

[53]   J. Zhang and L. Wang, "The emerging world of TCR-T cell trials against cancer: a systematic review," *Technology in cancer research & treatment,* vol. 18, p. 1533033819831068, 2019.

[54]   T. N. Schumacher, W. Scheper, and P. Kvistborg, "Cancer neoantigens," *Annual review of immunology,* vol. 37, pp. 173-200, 2019.

[55]   N. Bercovici, M.-T. Duffour, S. Agrawal, M. Salcedo, and J.-P. Abastado, "New methods for assessing T-cell responses," *Clinical and diagnostic laboratory immunology,* vol. 7, no. 6, p. 859, 2000.

[56]   R. Yossef *et al.,* "Enhanced detection of neoantigen-reactive T cells targeting unique and shared oncogenes for personalized cancer immunotherapy," *JCI insight,* vol. 3, no. 19, 2018.

[57]   L. Danilova *et al.,* "The mutation-associated neoantigen functional expansion of specific T cells (MANAFEST) assay: a sensitive platform for monitoring antitumor immunity," *Cancer immunology research,* vol. 6, no. 8, pp. 888-899, 2018.

[58]   L. De Moor *et al.,* "High-throughput fabrication of vascularized spheroids for bioprinting," *Biofabrication,* vol. 10, no. 3, p. 035009, 2018.

[59]   R. A. Wimmer *et al.,* "Human blood vessel organoids as a model of diabetic vasculopathy," *Nature,* vol. 565, no. 7740, pp. 505-510, 2019.

[60]   A. P. McGuigan and M. V. Sefton, "Vascularized organoid engineered by modular assembly enables blood perfusion," *PNAS,* vol. 103, no. 31, pp. 11461-11466, 2006.

[61]   M. W. Laschke and M. D. Menger, "Spheroids as vascularization units: From angiogenesis research to tissue engineering applications," *Biotechnology advances,* vol. 35, no. 6, pp. 782-791, 2017.

[62]   H. Lawall, P. Bramlage, and B. Amann, "Treatment of peripheral arterial disease using stem and progenitor cell therapy," *J. Vasc. Surg.,* vol. 53, no. 2, pp. 445-53, Feb 2011, doi: 10.1016/j.jvs.2010.08.060.

[63]   C. M. B. Botham, W. L.; Cooke, J. P., "Clinical trials of adult stem cell therapy for peripheral artery disease," *Methodist Debakey Cardiovasc. J.,* vol. 9, no. 4, 2013.

[64]   E. Benoit, T. F. O'Donnell, and A. N. Patel, "Safety and efficacy of autologous cell therapy in critical limb ischemia: a systematic review," *Cell Transplant.,* vol. 22, no. 3, pp. 545-62, 2013, doi: 10.3727/096368912X636777.

[65]   S. P. Cavnar, E. Salomonsson, K. E. Luker, G. D. Luker, and S. Takayama, "Transfer, imaging, and analysis plate for facile handling of 384 hanging drop 3D tissue spheroids," *J. Lab. Autom.,* vol. 19, no. 2, pp. 208-214, 2014.

[66]   J. M. Kelm *et al.,* "VEGF profiling and angiogenesis in human microtissues," *J. Biotechnol.,* vol. 118, no. 2, pp. 213-229, 2005.

[67] T. Liu, M. Winter, and B. Thierry, "Quasi-spherical microwells on superhydrophobic substrates for long term culture of multicellular spheroids and high throughput assays," *Biomaterials,* vol. 35, no. 23, pp. 6060-6068, 2014.

[68] J. M. Lee, L. Yang, E.-J. Kim, C. D. Ahrberg, K.-B. Lee, and B. G. Chung, "Generation of uniform-sized multicellular tumor spheroids using hydrogel microwells for advanced drug screening," *Sci Rep,* vol. 8, no. 1, p. 17145, 2018.

[69] G. S. Jeong, Y. No da, J. Lee, J. Yoon, S. Chung, and S. H. Lee, "Viscoelastic lithography for fabricating self-organizing soft micro-honeycomb structures with ultra-high aspect ratios," *Nat. Commun.,* vol. 7, p. 11269, 2016, doi: 10.1038/ncomms11269.

[70] E. M. Kim *et al.,* "Fabrication of core-shell spheroids as building blocks for engineering 3D complex vascularized tissue," *Acta Biomater.,* 2019.

[71] R. Tiruvannamalai Annamalai, A. Y. Rioja, A. J. Putnam, and J. P. Stegemann, "Vascular network formation by human microvascular endothelial cells in modular fibrin microtissues," *ACS Biomater Sci Eng.,* vol. 2, no. 11, pp. 1914-1925, 2016.

[72] E. C. Novosel, C. Kleinhans, and P. J. Kluger, "Vascularization is the key challenge in tissue engineering," *Adv Drug Deliv Rev,* vol. 63, no. 4-5, pp. 300-11, Apr 30 2011, doi: 10.1016/j.addr.2011.03.004.

[73] S. Dimmeler, S. Ding, T. A. Rando, and A. Trounson, "Translational strategies and challenges in regenerative medicine," *Nat Med,* vol. 20, no. 8, pp. 814-21, Aug 2014, doi: 10.1038/nm.3627.

[74] J. J. Kim, L. Hou, and N. F. Huang, "Vascularization of three-dimensional engineered tissues for regenerative medicine applications," *Acta Biomater,* vol. 41, pp. 17-26, Sep 1 2016, doi: 10.1016/j.actbio.2016.06.001.

[75] X. Sun, W. Altalhi, and S. S. Nunes, "Vascularization strategies of engineered tissues and their application in cardiac regeneration," *Adv Drug Deliv Rev,* vol. 96, pp. 183-94, Jan 15 2016, doi: 10.1016/j.addr.2015.06.001.

[76] M. Lovett, K. Lee, A. Edwards, and D. L. Kaplan, "Vascularization strategies for tissue engineering," *Tissue engineering. Part B, Reviews,* vol. 15, pp. 353-370, 2009, doi: 10.1089/ten.teb.2009.0085.

[77] B. M. Gillette *et al.,* "In situ collagen assembly for integrating microfabricated three-dimensional cell-seeded matrices," *Nat. Mater.,* vol. 7, no. 8, pp. 636-40, Aug 2008, doi: 10.1038/nmat2203.

[78] T. Goto *et al.,* "Search for appropriate experimental methods to create stable hind-limb ischemia in mouse," *Tokai J Exp Clin Med,* vol. 31, no. 3, pp. 128-132, 2006.

[79] A. Ponticorvo and A. K. Dunn, "How to build a Laser Speckle Contrast Imaging (LSCI) system to monitor blood flow," *Journal of visualized experiments: JoVE,* no. 45, 2010.

[80] D. A. Boas and A. K. Dunn, "Laser speckle contrast imaging in biomedical optics," *Journal of biomedical optics,* vol. 15, no. 1, p. 011109, 2010.

[81] B. M. Gillette, J. A. Jensen, M. Wang, J. Tchao, and S. K. Sia, "Dynamic hydrogels: switching of 3D microenvironments using two-component naturally derived extracellular matrices," *Adv Mater.,* vol. 22, no. 6, pp. 686-691, 2010.

[82] Y. X Chen, B. Cain, and P. Soman, "Gelatin methacrylate-alginate hydrogel with tunable viscoelastic properties," *AIMS Mater. Sci.,* vol. 4, no. 2, 2017.

[83] B. M. Gillette *et al.,* "Engineering extracellular matrix structure in 3D multiphase tissues," *Biomaterials,* vol. 32, no. 32, pp. 8067-76, Nov 2011, doi: 10.1016/j.biomaterials.2011.05.043.

[84] K. M. Wisdom *et al.*, "Matrix mechanical plasticity regulates cancer cell migration through confining microenvironments," *Nat Commun,* vol. 9, no. 1, p. 4144, Oct 8 2018, doi: 10.1038/s41467-018-06641-z.

[85] A. Prakasam, V. Maruthamuthu, and D. Leckband, "Similarities between heterophilic and homophilic cadherin adhesion," *Proceedings of the National Academy of Sciences,* vol. 103, no. 42, pp. 15434-15439, 2006.

[86] S. Gunti, A. T. Hoke, K. P. Vu, and N. R. London, "Organoid and spheroid tumor models: techniques and applications," *Cancers,* vol. 13, no. 4, p. 874, 2021.

[87] T. F. Goto, N.; Aki, A.; Kanabuchi, K.; Kimura, K.; Taira, H.; Tanaka, E.; Wakana, N.; Mori, H.; Inoue, H., "Search for appropriate experimental methods to create stable hind-limb ischemia in mouse," *Tokai J Exp Clin Med,* vol. 20, no. 31(3), pp. 128-32, 2006.

[88] T. Mirabella *et al.*, "3D-printed vascular networks direct therapeutic angiogenesis in ischaemia," *Nat. Biomed. Eng.,* vol. 1, no. 6, p. 0083, 2017, doi: 10.1038/s41551-017-0083.

[89] J. D. Briers, "Laser Doppler, speckle and related techniques for blood perfusion mapping and imaging," *Physiol. Meas.,* vol. 22, pp. R35-R66, 2001.

[90] J. P. Paques, "Alginate nanospheres prepared by internal or external gelation with nanoparticles," in *Microencapsulation and microspheres for food applications*: Elsevier, 2015, pp. 39-55.

[91] F. a. D. Administration, "Regulatory considerations for human cells, tissues, and cellular and tissue-based products: Minimal manipulation and homologous use; guidance for industry and food and drug administration staff; availability," *Federal Register,* vol. 82, no. 221, pp. 54290-54292, 2017.

[92] Y. Xing and K. A. Hogquist, "T-cell tolerance: central and peripheral," *Cold Spring Harbor perspectives in biology,* vol. 4, no. 6, p. a006957, 2012.

[93] D. Ganguly, S. Haak, V. Sisirak, and B. Reizis, "The role of dendritic cells in autoimmunity," *Nature Reviews Immunology,* vol. 13, no. 8, pp. 566-577, 2013.

[94] P. Bonaventura *et al.*, "Cold tumors: a therapeutic challenge for immunotherapy," *Frontiers in immunology,* vol. 10, p. 168, 2019.

[95] C. A. Klebanoff, S. A. Rosenberg, and N. P. Restifo, "Prospects for gene-engineered T cell immunotherapy for solid cancers," *Nature medicine,* vol. 22, no. 1, pp. 26-36, 2016.

[96] H.-I. Cho *et al.*, "A novel Epstein–Barr virus-latent membrane protein-1-specific T-cell receptor for TCR gene therapy," *British journal of cancer,* vol. 118, no. 4, pp. 534-545, 2018.

[97] M. D. Keller *et al.*, "SARS-CoV-2–specific T cells are rapidly expanded for therapeutic use and target conserved regions of the membrane protein," *Blood, The Journal of the American Society of Hematology,* vol. 136, no. 25, pp. 2905-2917, 2020.

[98] R. J. Creusot, M. Battaglia, M. G. Roncarolo, and C. G. Fathman, "Concise review: cell-based therapies and other non-traditional approaches for type 1 diabetes," *Stem Cells,* vol. 34, no. 4, pp. 809-819, 2016.

[99] M. J. Miller, A. S. Hejazi, S. H. Wei, M. D. Cahalan, and I. Parker, "T cell repertoire scanning is promoted by dynamic dendritic cell behavior and random T cell motility in the lymph node," *Proceedings of the National Academy of Sciences,* vol. 101, no. 4, pp. 998-1003, 2004.

[100] E. D'Ippolito, K. I. Wagner, and D. H. Busch, "Needle in a Haystack: The Naïve Repertoire as a Source of T Cell Receptors for Adoptive Therapy with Engineered T Cells," *International Journal of Molecular Sciences,* vol. 21, no. 21, p. 8324, 2020.

[101] C. Linnemann *et al.*, "High-throughput epitope discovery reveals frequent recognition of neo-antigens by CD4+ T cells in human melanoma," *Nature medicine,* vol. 21, no. 1, pp. 81-85, 2015.

[102] C. J. Cohen *et al.*, "Isolation of neoantigen-specific T cells from tumor and peripheral lymphocytes," *The Journal of clinical investigation,* vol. 125, no. 10, pp. 3981-3991, 2015.

[103] A. I. Segaliny *et al.*, "Functional TCR T cell screening using single-cell droplet microfluidics," *Lab on a Chip,* vol. 18, no. 24, pp. 3733-3749, 2018.

[104] M. A. Stockslager *et al.*, "Microfluidic platform for characterizing TCR–pMHC interactions," *Biomicrofluidics,* vol. 11, no. 6, p. 064103, 2017.

[105] V. M. Liarski *et al.*, "Quantifying in situ adaptive immune cell cognate interactions in humans," *Nature immunology,* vol. 20, no. 4, pp. 503-513, 2019.

[106] A. J. Walsh *et al.*, "Classification of T-cell activation via autofluorescence lifetime imaging," *Nature biomedical engineering,* vol. 5, no. 1, pp. 77-88, 2021.

[107] E. Strønen *et al.*, "Targeting of cancer neoantigens with donor-derived T cell receptor repertoires," *Science,* vol. 352, no. 6291, pp. 1337-1341, 2016.

[108] F. Kast, C. Klein, P. Umaña, A. Gros, and S. Gasser, "Advances in identification and selection of personalized neoantigen/T-cell pairs for autologous adoptive T cell therapies," *OncoImmunology,* vol. 10, no. 1, p. 1869389, 2021.

[109] F. C. Jammes and S. J. Maerkl, "How single-cell immunology is benefiting from microfluidic technologies," *Microsystems & Nanoengineering,* vol. 6, no. 1, pp. 1-14, 2020.

[110] S. Peng *et al.*, "Sensitive detection and analysis of neoantigen-specific T cell populations from tumors and blood," *Cell reports,* vol. 28, no. 10, pp. 2728-2738. e7, 2019.

[111] A. Gros *et al.*, "PD-1 identifies the patient-specific CD8+ tumor-reactive repertoire infiltrating human tumors," *The Journal of clinical investigation,* vol. 124, no. 5, pp. 2246-2259, 2014.

[112] M. Wolfl *et al.*, "Activation-induced expression of CD137 permits detection, isolation, and expansion of the full repertoire of CD8+ T cells responding to antigen without requiring knowledge of epitope specificities," *Blood, The Journal of the American Society of Hematology,* vol. 110, no. 1, pp. 201-210, 2007.

[113] Y. Simoni *et al.*, "Bystander CD8+ T cells are abundant and phenotypically distinct in human tumour infiltrates," *Nature,* vol. 557, no. 7706, pp. 575-579, 2018.

[114] A. M. Van der Leun, D. S. Thommen, and T. N. Schumacher, "CD8+ T cell states in human cancer: insights from single-cell analysis," *Nature Reviews Cancer,* vol. 20, no. 4, pp. 218-232, 2020.

[115] E. Moen, D. Bannon, T. Kudo, W. Graf, M. Covert, and D. Van Valen, "Deep learning for cellular image analysis," *Nature methods,* vol. 16, no. 12, pp. 1233-1246, 2019.

[116] W. Yu *et al.*, "Automatic classification of leukocytes using deep neural network," in *2017 IEEE 12th International Conference on ASIC (ASICON),* 2017: IEEE, pp. 1041-1044.

[117] A. Mencattini *et al.*, "Discovering the hidden messages within cell trajectories using a deep learning approach for in vitro evaluation of cancer drug treatments," *Scientific reports,* vol. 10, no. 1, pp. 1-11, 2020.

[118] C. L. Chen *et al.*, "Deep learning in label-free cell classification," *Scientific reports,* vol. 6, no. 1, pp. 1-16, 2016.

[119] S. E. Henrickson and U. H. von Andrian, "Single-cell dynamics of T-cell priming," *Current opinion in immunology,* vol. 19, no. 3, pp. 249-258, 2007.

[120] D. J. Zammit, L. S. Cauley, Q.-M. Pham, and L. Lefrançois, "Dendritic cells maximize the memory CD8 T cell response to infection," *Immunity,* vol. 22, no. 5, pp. 561-570, 2005.

[121] D. Zehn, S. Y. Lee, and M. J. Bevan, "Complete but curtailed T-cell response to very low-affinity antigen," *Nature,* vol. 458, no. 7235, pp. 211-214, 2009.

[122] S. M. Krummey *et al.*, "Low-affinity memory CD8+ T cells mediate robust heterologous immunity," *The Journal of Immunology,* vol. 196, no. 6, pp. 2838-2846, 2016.

[123] J. Schindelin *et al.*, "Fiji: an open-source platform for biological-image analysis," *Nature methods,* vol. 9, no. 7, pp. 676-682, 2012.

[124] C. Ocaña-Morgner, K. A. Wong, and A. Rodriguez, "Interactions between dendritic cells and CD4+ T cells during Plasmodium infection," *Malaria Journal,* vol. 7, no. 1, pp. 1-11, 2008.

[125] K. A. Hogquist, S. C. Jameson, W. R. Heath, J. L. Howard, M. J. Bevan, and F. R. Carbone, "T cell receptor antagonist peptides induce positive selection," *Cell,* vol. 76, no. 1, pp. 17-27, 1994.

[126] M. Cella, D. Scheidegger, K. Palmer-Lehmann, P. Lane, A. Lanzavecchia, and G. Alber, "Ligation of CD40 on dendritic cells triggers production of high levels of interleukin-12 and enhances T cell stimulatory capacity: TT help via APC activation," *The Journal of experimental medicine,* vol. 184, no. 2, pp. 747-752, 1996.

[127] K. Abdi, N. J. Singh, and P. Matzinger, "LPS Activated Dendritic cells:"Exhausted" or alert and waiting? DCs:"Exhausted", alerted or waiting?," *Journal of Immunology (Baltimore, Md.: 1950),* vol. 188, no. 12, p. 5981, 2012.

[128] P. Hermann, C. Van-Kooten, C. Gaillard, J. Banchereau, and D. Blanchard, "CD40 ligand-positive CD8+ T cell clones allow B cell growth and differentiation," *European journal of immunology,* vol. 25, no. 10, pp. 2972-2977, 1995.

[129] A. Scholer, S. Hugues, A. Boissonnas, L. Fetler, and S. Amigorena, "Intercellular adhesion molecule-1-dependent stable interactions between T cells and dendritic cells determine CD8+ T cell memory," *Immunity,* vol. 28, no. 2, pp. 258-270, 2008.

[130] H. D. Moreau, F. Lemaître, K. R. Garrod, Z. Garcia, A.-M. Lennon-Duménil, and P. Bousso, "Signal strength regulates antigen-mediated T-cell deceleration by distinct mechanisms to promote local exploration or arrest," *Proceedings of the National Academy of Sciences,* vol. 112, no. 39, pp. 12151-12156, 2015.

[131] R. R. Selvaraju, M. Cogswell, A. Das, R. Vedantam, D. Parikh, and D. Batra, "Grad-cam: Visual explanations from deep networks via gradient-based localization," in *Proceedings of the IEEE international conference on computer vision,* 2017, pp. 618-626.

[132] J. N. Mandl *et al.*, "Quantification of lymph node transit times reveals differences in antigen surveillance strategies of naive CD4+ and CD8+ T cells," *Proceedings of the National Academy of Sciences,* vol. 109, no. 44, pp. 18036-18041, 2012.

[133] M. Yarchoan, B. A. Johnson, E. R. Lutz, D. A. Laheru, and E. M. Jaffee, "Targeting neoantigens to augment antitumour immunity," *Nature Reviews Cancer,* vol. 17, no. 4, pp. 209-222, 2017.

[134] P. Hatfield *et al.*, "Optimization of dendritic cell loading with tumor cell lysates for cancer immunotherapy," *Journal of immunotherapy (Hagerstown, Md.: 1997),* vol. 31, no. 7, p. 620, 2008.

[135] G. Shakhar *et al.*, "Stable T cell–dendritic cell interactions precede the development of both tolerance and immunity in vivo," *Nature immunology,* vol. 6, no. 7, pp. 707-714, 2005.

[136] M. Arnaud, M. Duchamp, S. Bobisse, P. Renaud, G. Coukos, and A. Harari, "Biotechnologies to tackle the challenge of neoantigen identification," *Current opinion in biotechnology,* vol. 65, pp. 52-59, 2020.

[137] N. Varadarajan *et al.*, "A high-throughput single-cell analysis of human CD8+ T cell functions reveals discordance for cytokine secretion and cytolysis," *The Journal of clinical investigation,* vol. 121, no. 11, 2011.

[138] B. Dura *et al.*, "Profiling lymphocyte interactions at the single-cell level by microfluidic cell pairing," *Nature communications,* vol. 6, no. 1, pp. 1-13, 2015.

[139] M. Klinger *et al.*, "Multiplex identification of antigen-specific T cell receptors using a combination of immune assays and immune receptor sequencing," *PLoS One,* vol. 10, no. 10, p. e0141561, 2015.

[140] M. Ali *et al.*, "Induction of neoantigen-reactive T cells from healthy donors," *Nature protocols,* vol. 14, no. 6, pp. 1926-1943, 2019.

[141] A. V. Joglekar and G. Li, "T cell antigen discovery," *Nature Methods,* pp. 1-8, 2020.

[142] M. Bajénoff, N. Glaichenhaus, and R. N. Germain, "Fibroblastic reticular cells guide T lymphocyte entry into and migration within the splenic T cell zone," *The Journal of Immunology,* vol. 181, no. 6, pp. 3947-3954, 2008.

[143] W. Kastenmüller, M. Y. Gerner, and R. N. Germain, "The in situ dynamics of dendritic cell interactions," *European journal of immunology,* vol. 40, no. 8, pp. 2103-2106, 2010.

[144] M. F. Krummel, F. Bartumeus, and A. Gérard, "T cell migration, search strategies and mechanisms," *Nature Reviews Immunology,* vol. 16, no. 3, p. 193, 2016.

[145] P. Bousso and E. Robey, "Dynamics of CD8+ T cell priming by dendritic cells in intact lymph nodes," *Nature immunology,* vol. 4, no. 6, pp. 579-585, 2003.

[146] P. J. Attayek, S. A. Hunsucker, C. E. Sims, N. L. Allbritton, and P. M. Armistead, "Identification and isolation of antigen-specific cytotoxic T lymphocytes with an automated microraft sorting system," *Integrative Biology,* vol. 8, no. 12, pp. 1208-1220, 2016.

[147] P. M. Rosa, N. Gopalakrishnan, H. Ibrahim, M. Haug, and Ø. Halaas, "The intercell dynamics of T cells and dendritic cells in a lymph node-on-a-chip flow device," *Lab on a Chip,* vol. 16, no. 19, pp. 3728-3740, 2016.

[148] N. S. Lagali *et al.*, "Dendritic cell maturation in the corneal epithelium with onset of type 2 diabetes is associated with tumor necrosis factor receptor superfamily member 9," *Scientific reports,* vol. 8, no. 1, pp. 1-10, 2018.

[149] H. D. Moreau, G. Bogle, and P. Bousso, "A virtual lymph node model to dissect the requirements for T-cell activation by synapses and kinapses," *Immunology and cell biology,* vol. 94, no. 7, pp. 680-688, 2016.

[150] Y. Wang *et al.*, "Systematic prevention of bubble formation and accumulation for long-term culture of pancreatic islet cells in microfluidic device," *Biomedical microdevices,* vol. 14, no. 2, pp. 419-426, 2012.

[151] M. Sarmadi *et al.*, "Modeling, design, and machine learning-based framework for optimal injectability of microparticle-based drug formulations," *Science advances,* vol. 6, no. 28, p. eabb6594, 2020.

[152] D. B. Weibel, M. Kruithof, S. Potenta, S. K. Sia, A. Lee, and G. M. Whitesides, "Torque-actuated valves for microfluidics," *Analytical chemistry,* vol. 77, no. 15, pp. 4726-4733, 2005.

[153] M. A. Unger, H.-P. Chou, T. Thorsen, A. Scherer, and S. R. Quake, "Monolithic microfabricated valves and pumps by multilayer soft lithography," *Science,* vol. 288, no. 5463, pp. 113-116, 2000.

[154] P. B. Bach, S. A. Giralt, and L. B. Saltz, "FDA approval of tisagenlecleucel: promise and complexities of a $475 000 cancer drug," *Jama,* vol. 318, no. 19, pp. 1861-1862, 2017.

[155] Z. Aref, M. R. de Vries, and P. H. Quax, "Variations in surgical procedures for inducing hind limb ischemia in mice and the impact of these variations on neovascularization assessment," *International journal of molecular sciences,* vol. 20, no. 15, p. 3704, 2019.

[156] K. Kusamori *et al.*, "Transplantation of insulin-secreting multicellular spheroids for the treatment of type 1 diabetes in mice," *Journal of controlled release,* vol. 173, pp. 119-124, 2014.

[157] T. He, H. Mao, J. Guo, and Z. Yi, "Cell tracking using deep neural networks with multi-task learning," *Image and Vision Computing,* vol. 60, pp. 142-153, 2017.

[158] S. Lin *et al.*, "A flyover style microfluidic chip for highly purified magnetic cell separation," *Biosensors and Bioelectronics,* vol. 129, pp. 175-181, 2019.

[159] J. Krüger, K. Singh, A. O'Neill, C. Jackson, A. Morrison, and P. O'Brien, "Development of a microfluidic device for fluorescence activated cell sorting," *Journal of micromechanics and microengineering,* vol. 12, no. 4, p. 486, 2002.

[160] Y. Zhou *et al.*, "A microfluidic platform for trapping, releasing and super-resolution imaging of single cells," *Sensors and Actuators B: Chemical,* vol. 232, pp. 680-691, 2016.

[161] B. J. Nelson, I. K. Kaliakatsos, and J. J. Abbott, "Microrobots for minimally invasive medicine," *Annual review of biomedical engineering,* vol. 12, pp. 55-85, 2010.

[162] M. Sitti *et al.*, "Biomedical Applications of Untethered Mobile Milli/Microrobots," *Proceedings of the IEEE. Institute of Electrical and Electronics Engineers,* vol. 103, no. 2, pp. 205-224, 2015/02// 2015, doi: 10.1109/JPROC.2014.2385105.

[163] L. Ricotti *et al.*, "Biohybrid actuators for robotics: A review of devices actuated by living cells," *Science Robotics,* vol. 2, no. 12, p. eaaq0495, 2017.

[164] C. Hu, S. Pané, and B. J. Nelson, "Soft micro-and nanorobotics," *Annual Review of Control, Robotics, and Autonomous Systems,* vol. 1, pp. 53-75, 2018.

[165] R. G. Simmons, "Structured control for autonomous robots," *IEEE transactions on robotics and automation,* vol. 10, no. 1, pp. 34-43, 1994.

[166] M. Hoy, A. S. Matveev, and A. V. Savkin, "Algorithms for collision-free navigation of mobile robots in complex cluttered environments: a survey," *Robotica,* vol. 33, no. 3, pp. 463-497, 2015.

[167] K. J. Aström and R. M. Murray, *Feedback systems: an introduction for scientists and engineers.* Princeton university press, 2010.

[168] K. Lund *et al.*, "Molecular robots guided by prescriptive landscapes," *Nature,* vol. 465, no. 7295, p. 206, 2010.

[169] E. B. Steager, D. Wong, D. Mishra, R. Weiss, and V. Kumar, "Sensors for micro bio robots via synthetic biology," in *2014 IEEE International Conference on Robotics and Automation (ICRA),* 2014: IEEE, pp. 3783-3788.

[170] O. Ergeneman *et al.*, "In Vitro Oxygen Sensing Using Intraocular Microrobots," *IEEE Transactions on Biomedical Engineering,* vol. 59, no. 11, pp. 3104-3109, 2012/11// 2012, doi: 10.1109/TBME.2012.2216264.

[171] O. Ergeneman, G. Dogangil, M. P. Kummer, J. J. Abbott, M. K. Nazeeruddin, and B. J. Nelson, "A Magnetically Controlled Wireless Optical Oxygen Sensor for Intraocular Measurements," *IEEE Sensors Journal,* vol. 8, no. 1, pp. 29-37, 2008/01// 2008, doi: 10.1109/JSEN.2007.912552.

[172] W. Jing and D. J. Cappelleri, "Incorporating in-situ force sensing capabilities in a magnetic microrobot," in *2014 IEEE/RSJ International Conference on Intelligent Robots and Systems,* 2014/09// 2014, pp. 4704-4709, doi: 10.1109/IROS.2014.6943231. [Online]. Available: https://ieeexplore.ieee.org/document/6943231/?arnumber=6943231&tag=1

[173] T. Kawahara *et al.*, "On-chip microrobot for investigating the response of aquatic microorganisms to mechanical stimulation," (in en), *Lab on a Chip,* vol. 13, no. 6, pp. 1070-1078, 2013/02/20/ 2013, doi: 10.1039/C2LC41190C.

[174] L. Kong, J. Guan, and M. Pumera, "Micro- and nanorobots based sensing and biosensing," *Current Opinion in Electrochemistry,* vol. 10, pp. 174-182, 2018/08/01/ 2018, doi: 10.1016/j.coelec.2018.06.004.

[175] O. Ordeig, S. Y. Chin, S. Kim, P. V. Chitnis, and S. K. Sia, "An implantable compound-releasing capsule triggered on demand by ultrasound," *Scientific Reports,* vol. 6, 2016/03/11/ 2016, doi: 10.1038/srep22803.

[176] S. Fusco *et al.*, "An Integrated Microrobotic Platform for On-Demand, Targeted Therapeutic Interventions," *Advanced Materials,* vol. 26, no. 6, pp. 952-957, 2014 2014, doi: 10.1002/adma.201304098.

[177] S. Fusco *et al.*, "Shape-switching microrobots for medical applications: the influence of shape in drug delivery and locomotion," (in eng), *ACS applied materials & interfaces,* vol. 7, no. 12, pp. 6803-6811, 2015/04/01/ 2015, doi: 10.1021/acsami.5b00181.

[178] H. Ceylan, I. C. Yasa, O. Yasa, A. F. Tabak, J. Giltinan, and M. Sitti, "3D-Printed Biodegradable Microswimmer for Theranostic Cargo Delivery and Release," *ACS Nano,* vol. 13, no. 3, pp. 3353-3362, 2019/03/26/ 2019, doi: 10.1021/acsnano.8b09233.

[179] H. Li, G. Go, S. Y. Ko, J.-O. Park, and S. Park, "Magnetic actuated pH-responsive hydrogel-based soft micro-robot for targeted drug delivery," *Smart Materials and Structures,* vol. 25, no. 2, p. 027001, 2016.

[180] H. Lee, H. Choi, M. Lee, and P. Sukho, "Preliminary study on alginate/NIPAM hydrogel-based soft microrobot for controlled drug delivery using electromagnetic actuation and near-infrared stimulus," (in en), *Biomedical Microdevices,* vol. 20, no. 4, p. 103, 2018/11/16/ 2018, doi: 10.1007/s10544-018-0344-y.

[181] S. Lee *et al.*, "A Capsule-Type Microrobot with Pick-and-Drop Motion for Targeted Drug and Cell Delivery," (in eng), *Advanced Healthcare Materials,* vol. 7, no. 9, p. e1700985, 2018/05// 2018, doi: 10.1002/adhm.201700985.

[182] D. Jang, J. Jeong, H. Song, and S. K. Chung, "Targeted drug delivery technology using untethered microrobots: A review," *Journal of Micromechanics and Microengineering,* vol. 29, no. 5, p. 053002, 2019.

[183] J. Li *et al.*, "Development of a magnetic microrobot for carrying and delivering targeted cells," (in en), *Science Robotics,* vol. 3, no. 19, p. eaat8829, 2018/06/27/ 2018, doi: 10.1126/scirobotics.aat8829.

[184] S. Kim *et al.*, "Fabrication and characterization of magnetic microrobots for three-dimensional cell culture and targeted transportation," *Advanced Materials,* vol. 25, no. 41, pp. 5863-5868, 2013.

[185] G. Go *et al.*, "A Magnetically Actuated Microscaffold Containing Mesenchymal Stem Cells for Articular Cartilage Repair," *Advanced Healthcare Materials,* vol. 6, no. 13, p. 1601378, 2017/07/01/ 2017, doi: 10.1002/adhm.201601378.

[186] S. Jeon *et al.*, "Magnetically actuated microrobots as a platform for stem cell transplantation," *Science Robotics,* vol. 4, no. 30, p. eaav4317, 2019.

[187] K. Malachowski *et al.*, "Stimuli-Responsive Theragrippers for Chemomechanical Controlled Release," *Angewandte Chemie (International ed. in English),* vol. 53, no. 31, pp. 8045-8049, 2014/07/28/ 2014, doi: 10.1002/anie.201311047.

[188] H. Jia *et al.*, "Universal Soft Robotic Microgripper," *Small,* vol. 15, no. 4, p. 1803870, 2019, doi: 10.1002/smll.201803870.

[189] X. Wang, H. Huang, H. Liu, F. Rehfeldt, X. Wang, and K. Zhang, "Multi-Responsive Bilayer Hydrogel Actuators with Programmable and Precisely Tunable Motions," (in en), *Macromolecular Chemistry and Physics,* vol. 220, no. 6, p. 1800562, 2019 2019, doi: 10.1002/macp.201800562.

[190] J.-C. Kuo, H.-W. Huang, S.-W. Tung, and Y.-J. Yang, "A hydrogel-based intravascular microgripper manipulated using magnetic fields," *Sensors and Actuators A: Physical,* vol. 211, pp. 121-130, 2014/05/01/ 2014, doi: https://doi.org/10.1016/j.sna.2014.02.028.

[191] J. C. Breger *et al.*, "Self-Folding Thermo-Magnetically Responsive Soft Microgrippers," *ACS Applied Materials & Interfaces,* vol. 7, no. 5, pp. 3398-3405, 2015/02/11/ 2015, doi: 10.1021/am508621s.

[192] D. F. Williams, "On the mechanisms of biocompatibility," (in eng), *Biomaterials,* vol. 29, no. 20, pp. 2941-2953, 2008/07// 2008, doi: 10.1016/j.biomaterials.2008.04.023.

[193]   M. Kastellorizios, N. Tipnis, and D. J. Burgess, "Foreign Body Reaction to Subcutaneous Implants," J. D. Lambris, K. N. Ekdahl, D. Ricklin, and B. Nilsson, Eds., 2015 2015: Springer International Publishing, in Advances in Experimental Medicine and Biology, pp. 93-108.

[194] J. M. Anderson, "Biological Responses to Materials," *Annual Review of Materials Research,* vol. 31, no. 1, pp. 81-110, 2001, doi: 10.1146/annurev.matsci.31.1.81.

[195] J. M. Morais, F. Papadimitrakopoulos, and D. J. Burgess, "Biomaterials/Tissue Interactions: Possible Solutions to Overcome Foreign Body Response," *The AAPS Journal,* vol. 12, no. 2, pp. 188-196, 2010/02/09/ 2010, doi: 10.1208/s12248-010-9175-3.

[196] J. Li and D. J. Mooney, "Designing hydrogels for controlled drug delivery," *Nature reviews. Materials,* vol. 1, no. 12, 2016/12// 2016, doi: 10.1038/natrevmats.2016.71.

[197] R. Klopfleisch and F. Jung, "The pathology of the foreign body reaction against biomaterials," (in en), *Journal of Biomedical Materials Research Part A,* vol. 105, no. 3, pp. 927-940, 2017 2017, doi: 10.1002/jbm.a.35958.

[198] A. Vishwakarma *et al.*, "Engineering Immunomodulatory Biomaterials To Tune the Inflammatory Response," *Trends in Biotechnology,* vol. 34, no. 6, pp. 470-482, 2016/06/01/ 2016, doi: 10.1016/j.tibtech.2016.03.009.

[199] H. Yuk, B. Lu, and X. Zhao, "Hydrogel bioelectronics," (in en), *Chemical Society Reviews,* vol. 48, no. 6, pp. 1642-1667, 2019 2019, doi: 10.1039/C8CS00595H.

[200] J. Goding, C. Vallejo-Giraldo, O. Syed, and R. Green, "Considerations for hydrogel applications to neural bioelectronics," (in en), *Journal of Materials Chemistry B,* vol. 7, no. 10, pp. 1625-1636, 2019/03/06/ 2019, doi: 10.1039/C8TB02763C.

[201] R. Feiner and T. Dvir, "Tissue–electronics interfaces: From implantable devices to engineered tissues," *Nature Reviews Materials,* vol. 3, no. 1, p. 17076, 2018.

[202] K. C. Spencer, J. C. Sy, K. B. Ramadi, A. M. Graybiel, R. Langer, and M. J. Cima, "Characterization of Mechanically Matched Hydrogel Coatings to Improve the Biocompatibility of Neural Implants," (in En), *Scientific Reports,* vol. 7, no. 1, p. 1952, 2017/05/16/ 2017, doi: 10.1038/s41598-017-02107-2.

[203] A. A. Sharkawy, B. Klitzman, G. A. Truskey, and W. M. Reichert, "Engineering the tissue which encapsulates subcutaneous implants. I. Diffusion properties," (in en), *Journal of Biomedical Materials Research,* vol. 37, no. 3, pp. 401-412, 1997 1997, doi: 10.1002/(SICI)1097-4636(19971205)37:3<401::AID-JBM11>3.0.CO;2-E.

[204] W. K. Ward, E. P. Slobodzian, K. L. Tiekotter, and M. D. Wood, "The effect of microgeometry, implant thickness and polyurethane chemistry on the foreign body response to subcutaneous implants," *Biomaterials,* vol. 23, no. 21, pp. 4185-4192, 2002/11/01/ 2002, doi: 10.1016/S0142-9612(02)00160-6.

[205] E. R. Aurand, K. J. Lampe, and K. B. Bjugstad, "Defining and Designing Polymers and Hydrogels for Neural Tissue Engineering," *Neuroscience research,* vol. 72, no. 3, pp. 199-213, 2012/03// 2012, doi: 10.1016/j.neures.2011.12.005.

[206] J. L. Ifkovits, J. J. Devlin, G. Eng, T. P. Martens, G. Vunjak-Novakovic, and J. A. Burdick, "Biodegradable fibrous scaffolds with tunable properties formed from photo-cross-linkable poly (glycerol sebacate)," *ACS applied materials & interfaces,* vol. 1, no. 9, pp. 1878-1886, 2009.

[207] J. Kim, M. Dadsetan, S. Ameenuddin, A. J. Windebank, M. J. Yaszemski, and L. Lu, "In vivo biodegradation and biocompatibility of PEG/sebacic acid-based hydrogels using a cage implant system," *Journal of biomedical materials research Part A,* vol. 95, no. 1, pp. 191-197, 2010.

[208] O. Veiseh *et al.*, "Size- and shape-dependent foreign body immune response to materials implanted in rodents and non-human primates," (in eng), *Nature Materials,* vol. 14, no. 6, pp. 643-651, 2015/06// 2015, doi: 10.1038/nmat4290.

[209] B. Jang *et al.*, "Undulatory locomotion of magnetic multilink nanoswimmers," *Nano letters,* vol. 15, no. 7, pp. 4829-4833, 2015.

[210] M. Dai, R. Jungmann, and P. Yin, "Optical imaging of individual biomolecules in densely packed clusters," *Nature nanotechnology,* vol. 11, no. 9, p. 798, 2016.

[211] H. Wang and M. Pumera, "Fabrication of micro/nanoscale motors," *Chemical reviews,* vol. 115, no. 16, pp. 8704-8735, 2015.

[212] D. Asmar, M. Moussa, and J. Zelek, "On the role of machine learning algorithms in developing MEMS components," in *Proceedings International Conference on MEMS, NANO and Smart Systems,* 2003: IEEE, pp. 108-113.

[213]   Y. Jain, D. Chowdhury, and M. Chattopadhyay, "Machine Learning Based Fitness Tracker Platform Using MEMS Accelerometer," in *2017 International Conference on Computer, Electrical & Communication Engineering (ICCECE)*, 2017: IEEE, pp. 1-5.

[214]   M. L. Giger, "Machine learning in medical imaging," *Journal of the American College of Radiology,* vol. 15, no. 3, pp. 512-520, 2018.

[215]   J. Park, C. Jin, S. Lee, J. Y. Kim, and H. Choi, "Magnetically Actuated Degradable Microrobots for Actively Controlled Drug Release and Hyperthermia Therapy," *Advanced healthcare materials,* p. 1900213, 2019.

[216]   K. Kobayashi, C. Yoon, S. H. Oh, J. V. Pagaduan, and D. H. Gracias, "Biodegradable thermomagnetically responsive soft untethered grippers," *ACS applied materials & interfaces,* vol. 11, no. 1, pp. 151-159, 2018.

Appendix A: Soft medical microrobots: Design components and system integration

Medical microrobots are distinguished from other robotic systems in that they must function in the human body. As such, they exhibit special characteristics of size, function, and material choice. Recent advances have focused on fabrication techniques, locomotion at microscale environment, and targeted drug delivery. Here, we review these advances and examine related developments in material science and strategies for wireless control systems for communication, as well as data acquisition and processing. We focus on medical microrobots made of soft materials (with an emphasis on polymers and hydrogels), which are mechanically robust and deformable, offer tunable biophysical properties, and are highly biocompatible. Integration of the four design elements of locomotion, feedback and control, functionality, and biocompatibility (Fig A1) will be needed to develop a fully functioning medical microrobot with clinical utility in the human body, such as diagnostics and treatment of disease, maintenance of wellness, and improvement of overall performance.

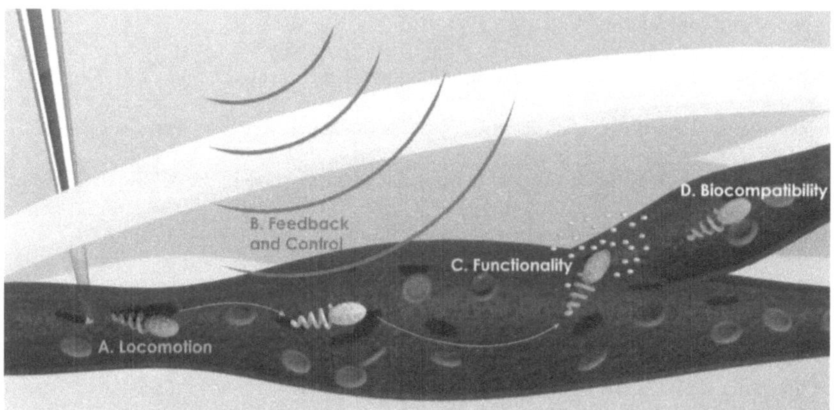

Figure A1: Design elements of a medical microrobot (MMR). An ideal MMR for implanted medical application must have (1) a method for moving from a given environment with minimal damage to surrounding features, whether if is fluid, soft tissue, or a boundary location; (2) responsiveness, so that it can adapt to real-time conditions, either by intrinsic controls based on physiological sensing or by extracorporeal control modalities, such as ultrasound or magnetism; (3) a sensing or intervention-oriented medical functionality, such as a drug or cell delivery; and (4) sufficient biocompatibility of materials to minimize any immune response and thereby maximize the life span of the device in vivo.

Design components

Locomotion

Mechanisms to enable locomotion of microrobots has been a focal point for researchers [161-163]. Microrobots must have sufficient propulsion force and dexterity to reach their intended application site. While macroscale devices are primarily affected by inertia or weight, microscale devices are influenced more by surface effects and viscous forces [161]. Previous reviews have classified designs for locomotion of microrobots (e.g. Nelson and co-workers noting actuated appendages, flexible joints, catalytic conversion of chemical energy, soft microrobots, stimuli-responsive movement [164]).

Feedback and control

MMRs must be responsive and adaptive once introduced into the human body; therefore, these devices must be controllable via a variety of possible modalities. Previous works have noted a need for wireless signals for the purpose of localization and tracking of the MMR [161]. In recent years, autonomous robots with well-developed control systems [165, 166] – from autonomous mobile robots in warehouses to unmanned aerial vehicles – have demonstrated a fundamental need for bidirectional signals (e.g. sensing information from robot to a controller, and functional signals from controller back to robot), with a robust method for signal processing in the controller (which could include machine-learning approaches). This paradigm of a feedback and control system [167], as applied for MMRs, is shown in Fig A2. Three different schemes are possible: a manually-controlled extracorporeal control system, an automated extracorporeal control system, and an automated internal control system. A primary consideration is the location of the controller, the element that processes signals from sensors, and sends instructions for locomotion or functionality back to the MMR. The controller can be either extracorporeal (outside the human body) or intrinsic (embedded within the MMR). Most approaches for MMRs rely on extracorporeal controllers as they are less constrained by space and power. Extracorporeal control is also versatile, allowing for manual intervention as well as machine-learning algorithms for closed-loop operation (i.e. automation of function of the MMR without manual intervention). On the other hand, MMRs with an intrinsic controller – functionally similar to a cell, microorganism, or organ – could be compact and autonomous. However, it is currently challenging to engineer MMRs with intrinsic control mechanisms beyond simple stimuli-responsive materials (possible approaches to engineer control mechanisms with complex logic include molecular machines [168] and synthetic biology [169]). Intrinsically controlled MMRs would also fall outside of mechanisms for manual intervention should it be required.

Common control modalities include magnetic, ultrasound, thermal, and optical mechanisms. When considering the appropriate control modality for a certain application, it is important to consider the needed range, depth of penetration, and resolution, as well as the capital equipment required. Furthermore, feedback and control mechanisms are crucial in minimizing any associated risks pertaining to MMRs, particularly by reducing likelihood of damage to surrounding tissue.

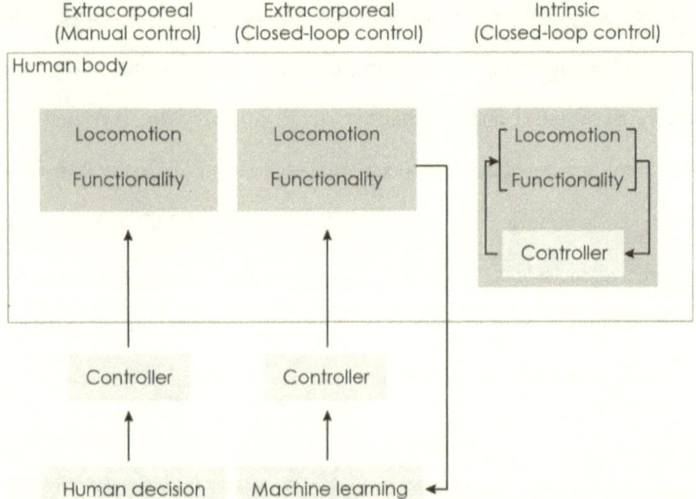

Figure A2. Mechanisms for feedback and control of a MMR. Three schemes are shown, with two involving a controller located outside the human body which can wirelessly receive and send signals to the MMR, and a third where the control mechanism is embedded within the MMR itself. A manual control mechanism allows for manual intervention and control, whereas an automated control mechanism (either one using machine-learning or one with an intrinsic controller) allows for autonomous operation. Note that the darker grey box represents the MMR.

Functionality

Upon reaching a target location, MMRs carry out a function in response to an extracorporeal or intrinsic trigger. In Table A1 we present specific requirements for MMRs depending on their intended functionality, such as sensing particular analytes in the surrounding environment, triggered delivery of small molecules or larger cargo such as cells, or microgripping to a tissue for surgical excision.

Table A1: Functionality. Description of commonly desired functions of a MMR. Depending on the intended functionality, the key parameters of a microrobot vary significantly.

	Important considerations	Examples
Sensing	Incorporation of receptor (to bind target analyte) and transducer (to convert the bio-recognition event into a signal that can be read out)	[170-174]
Delivery of drugs and small molecules	Sufficient drug loading (e.g. via encapsulation within hydrogel mesh or compartmentalization within device) *In vivo* drug stability	[175-182]
Delivery of cells	Sufficient cell loading (e.g. via encapsulation within porous hydrogel or compartmentalization within device) Maintenance of cell viability	[176, 181, 183-186]
Gripping	Mechanical robustness to ensure that the device does not deform or fracture while gripping the target	[187-191]

Biocompatibility

Finally, since MMRs may be in contact with biological fluids or tissue for potentially long time periods during *in vivo* applications, it is critical that they are biocompatible. In one definition of biocompatibility, the devices should carry out a specific application, with an appropriate host response [192]. Biological responses to implants initially consist of inflammatory and wound healing responses, but in the presence of a foreign body which cannot be phagocytosed by macrophages (devices <10um), wound healing evolves into a foreign body reaction (FBR), in which macrophages and monocytes fuse to form foreign body giant cells, and is followed by fibrous encapsulation of the foreign body [193, 194]. This can have significant unintended consequences, such as compromised patient safety (biosafety), and compromised device functionality (biofunctionality) [195]. However, as demonstrated in other fields such as tissue engineering [196-198] and bio-electronics [199, 200], the severity of the FBR, which is typically measured by the extent of fibrous encapsulation, can be modulated through careful device material selection and design. Specifically, the use of soft materials, with carefully tuned material properties, can enable device functionality for the intended duration, without causing harm to the patient. In Table A2 we discuss how material properties, as well as device properties can be leveraged to further modulate the FBR, thereby increasing the overall biocompatibility of

the MMR. The design of soft MMR's can also apply much of the research from tissue

engineering or bioelectronics to develop biocompatible soft implants at the microscale.

Table A2: Biocompatibility. Description of the effect of material and device properties (stiffness, porosity, biodegradability, geometry and size) on fibrotic scarring of implanted device, and the resulting effect of scarring on device functionality. These material and device properties can be tuned to maximize biocompatibility, and maintain device functionality.

Property of material or device	Effect on scarring		Impact of scarring on functionality	Reference
	Increased	Decreased		
Stiffness	Stiff	Soft	Higher electrical impedance across a tissue interface due to increased scarring from stiff neural electrodes results in reduced recording and stimulation efficiency	[199, 201, 202]
Porosity	Nonporous (more dense)	Porous (less dense)	Reduced diffusivity of analyte to be sensed or released cargo	[203, 204]
Biodegradability	Non-biodegradable or slowly degrading	Biodegradable or fast degrading	Reduced mass transfer between implants and surrounding tissue	[205-207]
Geometry and size	Small sphere (0.5 mm diameter, alginate)	Large sphere (1.5 mm diameter, alginate)	Reduced duration of control by encapsulated islet cells over blood glucose levels	[208]
	Large cylinder (2 mm diameter, polyurethane)	Small cylinder (0.3 mm diameter, polyurethane)	No specifically demonstrated impact on functionality	[204]

System integration

Many studies have demonstrated proof of concept of individual design components. However,

reaching *in vivo* impact will require integration of four different design elements, as reflected by

appropriate device geometry to achieve locomotion through target environments, responsiveness

to a relevant control modality, ability to perform specific functionalities at target sites, and

appropriate biocompatibility over the duration of use. (Table A3). Prior works in these four areas

have emphasized the following solutions. Methods for locomotion have included bio-inspired

designs, namely microswimmers which mimic bacteria, but this design exhibits limited capacities in terms of payload size and ability to maneuver outside of a purely fluid environment. For feedback and control, most demonstrations with externally-controlled modalities employ magnetic methods, including electromagnetic coils from a custom or MRI system and permanent magnets; typically, the corresponding implanted MMRs have embedded magnetic NPs, to ensure responsiveness. For functionality, while MMRs have been proposed as potential treatment options for a variety of conditions, the field thus far has largely emphasized methods of drug delivery. Finally, for biocompatibility, a large array of MMRs are fabricated from rigid materials and incorporate non-biocompatible magnetic nanoparticle, thereby increasing the likelihood of a fibrotic tissue response that will negate the device's functionality and locomotion principles. Hence, concepts towards integrated MMRs have exhibited one or more limitations, such as settings for locomotion (only one type of tissue, or behavior in swarm settings), depth and range of control mechanisms, biocompatibility, and biodegradability [209-211]. Very few MMRs have thus far fully integrated control, movement, and medical functionality, particularly for *in vivo* contexts.

Future perspectives and conclusion

From recent research across multiple design elements, a coherent paradigm for how to build an integrated MMR is emerging. At the moment, emphasis has been placed on locomotion and drug-delivery functions. For materials, in addition to microelectronics and biohybrid designs, soft materials are increasingly being developed and shaped for novel uses. In the future, to achieve precise operation, wireless communication modalities will be increasingly integrated into MMRs as part of well-developed feedback and control systems – for data acquisition, communication, and control – as seen in increasingly prevalent macroscale robotic systems. On the other hand, unlike macroscale robotic systems, by virtue of the human body environment as well as constraints placed on the size and power of the communications elements, the wireless communication modalities will likely be different.

Another likely trend is increasing incorporation of machine learning, such that the devices can "learn" from an environment [212], which can lead to closed-loop operation and increasing autonomous behavior. An early demonstration is a MEMS circuit that senses shear stress, analyzes the signal via neural network, and then reduces the drag of the device by adjusting micro-actuators [212]. More recently, MEMS devices, namely gyroscopes and accelerometers, have become commonplace consumer products; integration of machine learning with such wearable devices enables additional training functionalities, such as for predicting risk factors for obesity based on daily calorie and step count [213]. In addition, machine learning has begun to assist in radiological imaging tasks, such as detection, diagnosis, and therapeutic response [214]. In the future, integration of machine learning with implantable devices and microrobots is likely to become increasingly relevant to achieve unprecedented functions.

With such recent research and emerging trends, the tantalizing but technically demanding vision of MMRs is coming closer. Successful development of MMRs could enable a medical future with minimally invasive interventions (and corresponding reductions in risk of infection, recovery time, pain, and other complications), and novel approaches for maintenance of wellness and improvement in overall human performance.

Device	Material	Fabrication Method	Locomotion		Controller mechanism	Functionality	Biocompatibility tests	Reference
			Geometry	Intended location				
Biodegradable microswimmer	Gelatin methacryloyl (matrix metalloproteinase 2 (MMP2)-responsive) with iron oxide NPs	3D printing via two photon polymerization	Cylindrical core wrapped by double helix, with cones at the ends	Tumor site	Extracorporeal (magnetic modality) Intrinsic (sensing of MMP2 levels)	Sensing (MMP2 levels) Delivery of drugs (targeted release of drugs and NPs coated with antibodies to tag tumor cells)	*In vitro* cytotoxicity (co-culture of microswimmer degradation products with cancer cell line for 24 hours)	[178]
Foldable bilayer microgripper	pNIPAAM (thermoresponsive) with multiwall carbon nanotubes and iron oxide NPs	Soft lithography	Horseshoe-like	Through blood vessels	Extracorporeal (AC and DC magnetic modality)	Gripping of tissue (targeted opening or closing of grippers to pick up or release blood clot)	None	[190]
Foldable bilayer with internal compartment	Poly (2-hydroxyethyl methacrylate) (pH-responsive) and polyethylene glycol diacrylate (PEGDA) with iron oxide NPs	Photolithography	Sphere-like	Through blood vessels, to tumor site	Extracorporeal (magnetic modality) Intrinsic (sensing of pH levels)	Sensing (pH levels) Delivery of drugs (targeted release of microbeads loaded with an anti-cancer drug)	*In vitro* cytotoxicity (co-culture of microrobots with cancer cell line for 24 hours)	[179]
Degradable hyperthermia microrobot	PEGDA and pentaerythritol with iron oxide NPs	Two photon polymerization	Helical	Tumor site	Extracorporeal (rotating and alternating magnetic modality)	Drug delivery (targeted release of anticancer drug) Thermal ablation	*In vitro* cytotoxicity (co-culture of microrobots (without anticancer drug) with cancer cell line for 48 hours)	[215]

Foldable bilayer with internal compartment	PEGDA and pNIPAAM-graphene oxide nanocomposite (thermoresponsive) with alginate microparticles encapsulating iron oxide NPs	Photolithography	Sphere-like (jellyfish- or Venus fly trap-like structures)	Remote parts of the body (e.g. hepatic artery)	Extracorporeal (magnetic modality) Extracorporeal (NIR modality)	Drug or cell delivery (targeted release of alginate microparticles encapsulating cells or drugs)	*In vitro* cytotoxicity (co-culture of hydrogel bilayers or hydrogel-conditioned medium with fibroblasts for 2 days) *In vitro* viability of encapsulated mesenchymal stem cells for 7 days	[176]
Biodegradable foldable bilayer grippers	Poly(oligoethylene glycol methyl ether methacrylate (M_n = 500)-bis(2-methacryloyl)oxyethyl disulfide) (thermoresponsive) and poly(acrylamide-N,N'-bis(acyloyl)cystamine) with iron oxide NPs	Photolithography	Sphere-like	Through tissue	Extracorporeal (magnetic modality) Intrinsic (sensing of temperature)	Sensing (temperature) Gripping of tissue (targeted closing of grippers to excise cells)	*In vitro* cytotoxicity (co-culture of grippers with endothelial cell line for 3 days)	[216]

Table A3: **Integration of hydrogel-based MMRs.** Examples of integrated soft MMRs which satisfy all four of the design characteristics of movement, control, functionality, and biocompatibility. All of these devices are at least partially magnetically controlled. Future diversity in control modalities could expand the range of functionalities and overcome some of the listed limitations.